HANDBOOK ON
CRITICAL LIFE ISSUES

Pope John Center
Task Force on Critical Life Issues

Raymond J. Adamek, Ph.D.
Professor of Sociology
Kent State University, Kent, OH

The Reverend Lorenzo Albacete, S.T.D. (Cand.)
Assistant for Theological Matters
Washington, DC

Paul W. Armstrong, J.D., LL.M.
Counsellor at Law
Morristown, NJ

The Reverend Benedict M. Ashley, O.P., Ph.D., S.T.M.
Professor of Moral Theology
Aquinas Institute of Theology,
St. Louis, MO

James Bopp, Jr., J.D.
Attorney, General Counsel
National Right-to-Life Committee
Washington, DC

The Reverend Robert A. Brungs, S.J., S.T.L., Ph.D.
Director
Institute for Theological Encounter
with Science and Technology
St. Louis, MO

The Reverend Frank X. Cleary, S.J., S.S.L., S.T.D.
Associate Professor of Scripture
St. Louis University, St. Louis, MO

John E. Codd, M.D.
Director, Transplant Service
St. Louis University Hospital,
St. Louis, MO

†The Reverend John R. Connery, S.J., S.T.D.
Professor of Moral Theology
Loyola University, Chicago, IL

John F. Cross, Ph.D.
Associate Professor of Psychology
St. Louis University, St. Louis, MO

The Reverend James J. Doyle, C.S.C., S.T.L., M.A.
Professor of Theology
King's College, Wilkes Barre, PA

Mari Anne Hamilton, J.D.
Legal Consultant
U.S. Department of Health and
Human Services
Washington, DC

†Dennis J. Horan, J.D.
Attorney at Law
Chicago, IL

Sister Margaret John Kelly, D.C., Ph.D.
Vice President, Division of Mission
Services
Catholic Health Association of the
U.S.
St. Louis, MO

Micheline M. Mathews-Roth, B.S., M.D.
Principal Research Associate in
Medicine
Harvard University School of
Medicine
Cambridge, MA

The Reverend Albert S. Moraczewski, O.P., Ph.D.
Regional Director—Houston office
Houston, TX

The Reverend Robert A. Patterson, M.Div.
Director, Pastoral Service
Catholic Health Association of the
U.S.
St. Louis, MO

M. Waheed-uz-Zaman Rana, Ph.D.
Associate Professor of Anatomy
St. Louis University School of
Medicine
St. Louis, MO

Robert S. Rosenthal, J.D., M.S.
Attorney at Law
St. Louis, MO

J. Stuart Showalter, J.D., M.F.S.
Director, Division of Legal Services
Catholic Health Association of the
U.S.
St. Louis, MO

Sister Clara Ternes, A.S.C., R.N., M.A.
Director, A.S.C. Health Ministries
St. Louis, MO

The Reverend Granger E. Westberg, D.D.
Adjunct Professor
College of Medicine, University of
Illinois
Chicago, IL

HANDBOOK ON CRITICAL LIFE ISSUES

REVISED EDITION

Edited and revised by: Donald G. McCarthy, Ph.D.,
Edward J. Bayer, S.T.D.

Pope John Center

Braintree, Massachusetts

Nihil Obstat:
  Reverend James A. O'Donohoe, J.C.D.
    Censor Deputatus

Imprimatur:
  Bernard Cardinal Law, Archdiocese of Boston, January 23, 1989
The Nihil Obstat and Imprimatur are a declaration that a book or pamphlet is considered to be free from doctrinal or moral error. It is not implied that those who have granted the Nihil Obstat and Imprimatur agree with the contents, opinions, or statements expressed.

Copyright, 1st edition, 1982 and revised edition, 1988
by
The Pope John XXIII Medical-Moral
Research and Education Center
186 Forbes Road
Braintree, Massachusetts 02184

6th Printing, (revised edition)

This revised edition is dedicated to the memory of two recently deceased members of the original Task Force on Critical Life Issues: Reverend John R. Connery, S.J., and Mr. Dennis J. Horan, J.D.

These two dedicated professionals—one a priest, a Jesuit and eminent moralist, the other a husband, father and outstanding lawyer—were a living example of the vocation of the whole Church, people and pastors, working with their own unique gifts so that human beings may be treated with the gentle and strong compassion of Christ.

Library of Congress Cataloging in Publication Data
Main entry under title:

A Handbook on critical life issues, revised edition

Handbook on critical life issues / edited and revised by Donald G.
  McCarthy, Edward J. Bayer. — Rev. ed.
      p. cm.
    Bibliography: p.
    Includes index.
    ISBN (invalid) 0–935372–24–5 (pbk.) : $9.95
      1. Medical ethics. 2. Bioethics. 3. Medical care—Law and
  legislation. I. McCarthy, Donald G. II. Bayer, Edward J., 1930–
R724.H23 1988
174'.2—dc19   88–38958
                                                             CIP

Table of Contents

Preface to the
Revised Edition

The editors and contributors of the original edition wish to express their gratitude to theologian confreres, reviewers, physicians, nurses, hospital administrators, teachers, students, and all who have given attention to the first edition of this work. We are grateful, particularly, to Mrs. Jeanne L. Burke who navigated the text through months of preparation. Helpful comments, as well as medical, legal, and theological developments since that edition was published, have indicated the usefulness of some revision.

In particular, the following seem to merit an updated attention:

—certain theological considerations of therapeutic abortion in the strictest sense (when otherwise both mother and child will die shortly);
—the "selective reduction" of the number of fetuses a woman is carrying as a result of in vitro fertilization;
—new efforts to avoid impregnation from rape;
—expanded techniques of organ "harvesting" of human tissues and organs from embryos and fetuses for therapeutic or experimental purposes;
—debates within the Church and in society at large regarding the prolonging of the life of the seriously sick or handicapped;
—some judicial and legal developments affecting this latter issue.

The editors can hope only that this present revision will be as useful to its readers as the previous edition seems to have been.

Donald G. McCarthy
Edward J. Bayer

August 4, 1988

PART ONE

Persons: Priceless and Vulnerable

Preview of Chapter 1

- Science could make possible new life forms like clones and animal/human hybrids. What is really distinctive about being a human person?

- Psychology studies the human personality by studying its traits or characteristics. But persons cannot be understood very adequately this way.

- Philosophy has both an objective and a subjective approach to describing what persons are.

- Human persons must be seen in terms, not only of their unique kind of knowledge and their creative freedom, but also of their unique kind of existence—the ontological mystery.

- Fathers Ashley and O'Rourke propose a simple modern description of the human person as "embodied intelligent freedom."

- Persons cannot exist apart from community; the Christian vision of the person can be a leaven in the pluralistic society of the United States.

CHAPTER 1

The Person as Known by Reason and Reflection

The movie "Boys From Brazil" raised in popular entertainment the startling possibility of "xeroxing" people. The plot revolved around the as yet untried scientific technique of generating human "clones," individuals who are carbon copies of a single adult.

The word "clone" has entered our vocabulary. People who are concerned about ethical values and norms (we will call them ethicists in this book) wonder about the ethical or moral aspects of cloning. But, knowing human curiosity about the unknown and the willingness to "try anything once," it seems safe to predict that, if cloning ever becomes feasible, some scientist *somewhere* will try it. One report of human cloning actually done already was probably a hoax.

But science fiction, long before "Star Wars," was filled with robots and Frankenstein's monsters. *Scientists seem to have a strong urge to manufacture robot human beings by a technological procedure.* No doubt the ultimate scientific benefit would be quality control of the product. When human parents come together in conjugal love, they have no guarantee of actually procreating a child, to say nothing of "quality control" of their offspring.

Just over the horizon beyond cloning another scientific challenge lies in wait: animal/human hybrids. Up until now, mermaids swam around only in books. But future science may unite the genetic material for a young lady with that of a dolphin. The possibilities are mind-boggling and terribly disturbing.

A hybrid union of a monkey and a human being may not seem as outlandish as the dolphin mermaid. In fact, a hundred years ago when Charles Darwin's research on evolution first gripped the public fantasy, some people thought that human persons and monkeys weren't all that different. It almost seemed to some that the major difference was in the size of the brain and the skull cavity.

But the difference between humans and the most advanced monkey or chimpanzee goes far deeper than the number of brain cells. Some years ago a chimpanzee named Sarah was featured in *Scientific American* because she had a "vocabulary" of some 130 "words" based on variously shaped and colored pieces of plastic.[1] But Sarah hasn't written any poems or made any free decisions or even talked back to her trainer. Human persons *are* different from animals, they even write books like this one.

Yet human persons are also very different from one another. Contrast a cannibal in the South Pacific with a Wall Street businessman in a grey flannel suit. The businessman might take his wife *out to* lunch and the cannibal might have his wife *for* lunch!

Scholars who study cultural and ethnic differences between people often hint that people are so different that there is no common human nature. One might say that the only thing common about people is that they are all different.

That is not true. Humans are different from animals. And that very difference is shared in common by all human persons. Despite cultural differences, all human persons are able to "humanize" their own lives, or to adapt to their surroundings through the human gifts of knowledge and freedom. Fathers Ashley and O'Rourke, two Catholic ethicists, have discussed this question. *"Culture,"* they wrote, *is only the expression of our nature, which is to be intelligently free."*[2]

---

[1] *An Ethical Evaluation of Fetal Experimentation: An Interdisciplinary Study,* edited by Donald McCarthy and Albert Moraczewski, O.P. (St. Louis, Mo: The Pope John Center, 1976), p. 23.

[2] Ashley, Benedict M. and O'Rourke, Kevin D., *Health Care Ethics.* A Theological Analysis (St. Louis, Mo.: The Catholic Health Association, 2nd Edit, 1982), p. 4.

4

So the Wall Street businessman and the cannibal in the South Pacific are both human persons. In Parts II and III this volume will discuss specific and critical issues involving the life and death of human persons. For instance, the last chapter of this book talks about determining by brain criteria whether death has taken place. But what is death?

Human death is the end of life as we know it. But what is human life? Is it the same as the life of a human *person*? If it is, what is a human person? The questions of cloning, mermaids, and chimpanzees all come up in deciding what is a person. The rest of this chapter will reflect on what human reason can tell us about being a person.

The other chapters in Part I of this volume will continue the study of human persons, ending in Chapter 6 with the common human experience of suffering.

Persons and Personalities

Being a human person means having one's own "personality." That word sometimes refers to special people, celebrities. Sports personalities, television personalities, political personalities are all people in the public's eye.

Sometimes the pressures of public attention affect people's personalities. Guillermo Vilas, the famous Argentine tennis star, once said that, "It's not the person who changes, but the persons who surround him." He gave a picturesque example. "My parents have become so conditioned to reacting for the benefit of local newsmen and television cameras," he said, "that they smile when the light goes on in the refrigerator at home!"

But, even without public attention, everyone has a personality. The science of psychology studies human personality, which it understands as the sum of the unique psychological qualities which influence the behavior of each person. A variety of theories are used to explain how an individual's actual life experiences interact with inherited potential to shape his or her personality.

Much psychological research has concentrated on personality traits. One kind of research tries to determine what are the relationships between behavior and factors or traits shared by all individuals or at least by identifiable subgroups of people.

In this approach one might begin by assuming that all people have certain common traits but in different degrees. Research then attempts to measure these traits in given individuals and establish the relationship between the trait itself and behavior that would show the trait. If the relationship is strong, knowledge of an individual's personality traits would predict how that person will actually behave in given situations. But, in fact, research shows a weak relationship as a rule.[3] _Personality traits do not predict the behavior of even most of the people most of the time._

Another kind of psychological research has sought to investigate whether personality traits remain stable over substantial periods in the life of individual persons. This is called the longitudinal method. Relatively few studies have been done. One study showed that specific personality characteristics did not usually remain constant from adolescence to adulthood. For example, while achievement and I.Q. remained moderately stable, expressions of sexual interests, hostility, impulsiveness, power orientation, morals, fantasizing, and competitiveness showed no pronounced stability. Another study tended to support this one.[4]

Another approach to personality study was popularized by the well-known Gordon Allport. He sought to discover which traits were relevant to individual persons from their own perspective. He held that each trait is unique in the way it functions within a person's total makeup. Allport believed his research to show that in their behavior different people are not all consistent in the same way, but that they tend to be consistent with themselves.

Obviously, the research described here is only a tiny fraction of all that has been done. _But it does seem that human persons cannot be readily reduced to bundles of traits which blindly produce behavior much as a press prints a newspaper._ What does make people tick? Philosophy, the reflective study of the human world and its meaning, has been asking this question for all of recorded history.

Philosophy and Human Persons

Some philosophers, especially in the period of ancient Greek philosophy and its medieval versions in the 13th century, looked at human persons as individuals, each possessing the same kind of existence or reality. Aristotle, for example, considered human persons to be "rational animals." They belong to the genus or general classification of animals with rationality as a special quality distinguishing them from other animals.

Boethius, a philosopher of the sixth century A.D., used this definition of a person: An individual substance of a rational nature. Great

---

[3]Zimbardo, Philip G., _Psychology and Life_ (Glenview, IL., Scot, Foresman Publ., 1979), p. 470.
[4]_Ibid_, p. 471.

medieval philosophers like St. Thomas Aquinas carried forward this objective view of human persons as members of the human species. *In this view, to be a person means to be a particular kind of living being, despite the individual and cultural differences mentioned above between the cannibal and the Wall Street businessman.*

Beginning after the Middle Ages with the work of René Descartes (1596–1650), a more subjective view of the human person emerges. In this approach, the philosopher begins with his or her own self-awareness of the world as appearing in thought and reflection. The emphasis now rests on thought (for Descartes, *cogito ergo sum*. I think, therefore I am). Others are recognized as persons when they, too, manifest indications of similar conscious experience.

This latter approach to understanding human persons has dominated much of the philosophical world since the 17th century. Great thinkers like Kant, Hegel, and, in the 20th century, Edmund Husserl, have followed this approach. It has led to many philosophical puzzles. Among them are the relationship of mind and matter; the problem of how one self can really *know* another self; and the nagging thought that perhaps the real world is altogether different from the world as it appears.

In the world of Catholic philosophy, a strong 20th century movement called Neo-Thomism has taken shape. It features a re-discovery and a modern interpretation of the wisdom of St. Thomas Aquinas and the philosophers of his tradition. Well-known philosophers like Jacques Maritain and Etienne Gilson argued that human knowledge is unequivocally realistic, in contact with objective reality. They rejected the narrow starting point of subjective consciousness used by Descartes and so many others.

Since the Second World War, another approach to the human person has emerged. Here the emphasis is laid on freedom rather than self-consciousness. Jean Paul Sartre took an extreme and atheistic position by holding that in freedom human persons create themselves and give meaning to an otherwise meaningless and absurd world.

Other philosophers of human freedom like Soren Kierkegaard, Gabriel Marcel, and Emmanuel Mounier, understand freedom as a gift of God to be used in searching for Him. Out of this reflection comes a view of human persons as independent beings with a spiritual nature which transcends the limits of purely biological and material reality. Mounier spoke of "substance" and "independence in being" in describing human persons. *These philosophers stress that each person freely creates his or her personality but can also discover and freely accept a relationship with the Supreme Person whom Marcel called the "Absolute Thou."*

Yet each human person, in this contemporary approach, retains an essential social relationship with other human persons. The person is related to other persons as a free moral agent uniting with other agents in pursuing the common good. This view, then, rejects both the collectivism of Marxist theories of society and the extreme individualism of authors like Herbert Spencer who believe that political society exists merely to allow individuals to pursue their private interests alone.

Obviously, this brief overview of the way some philosophers have viewed the human person only touched briefly the major points of difference and development. But it offers background now for a contemporary description of human persons in accord with the Judeo-Christian tradition and Catholic teaching.

Person and Mystery

Clearly, no one can define human persons with the kind of simplicity and completeness with which the mathematician defines a triangle. The vastly different ways philosophers have approached the subject of their own personhood indicates the complexity of the task.

The document of the Second Vatican Council of the Catholic Church in 1965 which described human persons noted this very diversity:

> What is man? He has put forward, and continues to put forward, many views about himself, views that are divergent and even contradictory. Often he either sets himself up as the absolute measure of all things, or debases himself to the point of despair.[5]

The twin emphases in modern philosophy on the self-consciousness of the person and the person's self-creating freedom indicate primary and inescapable truths about personhood. Yet, the older view of persons as independent living substances cannot be overlooked, either.

The Catholic tradition in philosophical reflection, both in the Middle Ages and in the 20th century Neo-Thomism, insists on the understanding of persons as individual bodily agents gifted with knowledge and freedom. This view of the person can exist comfortably with—and even enrich—modern evolutionary theories which indicate that persons change and develop culturally and individually.

The document of the Second Vatican Council mentioned above highlighted the particular kind of existence human persons experience:

---

[5]*The Church in the Modern World (Gaudium et Spes)* #12.

8

> Man, though made of body and soul, is a unity. Through his very bodily condition he sums up in himself the elements of the natural world. Through him they are thus brought to their highest perfection and can raise their voice in praise freely given to the creator . . .
>
> Man is not deceived when he regards himself as superior to bodily things and as more than just a speck of nature or a nameless unit in the city of man. For by his power to know himself in the depths of his being he rises above the whole universe of mere objects.[6]

In its description of human persons this Catholic document begins, as indicated here, with human bodily existence. Then it moves on, not only to self-conscious knowledge, but to the power of the mind to achieve spiritual knowledge and wisdom. The description climaxes with the gift of moral conscience and the human freedom with which persons pursue the good.[7]

Fathers Ashley and O'Rourke, in the study mentioned above, insist that human persons and human beings are one and the same. Human persons are bodily beings, evolving perhaps out of the natural world, but never separated from it. "Consequently, human self-awareness and freedom emerge," they write, "only at high points of a very complex process, much of which is subconscious and part of the determinism of nature." They insist, along with much of recent philosophy, that bodily identity is necessary to the notion of the human person. *Their simplified description of the person is "embodied intelligent freedom."*[8]

Such simple phrases to describe human persons may suggest that philosophy has not progressed much beyond the "rational animal" description of persons used by Aristotle. It has, and it hasn't. The understanding of the world of nature has surely developed radically since the days of the Greeks. But human persons are still human persons!

Perhaps the single predominant theme in philosophical reflection about persons in the past 300 years has been the pervasive skepticism about the person as a being-in-the-world. This is linked with the subjectivism described above. Neo-Thomism has sought to overcome that skepticism. So have personalist philosophers like Gabriel Marcel.

In 1933, Marcel wrote a profound essay titled, "On the Ontological Mystery." He reflected on the human experience of love, hope, creative

---

[6]*Ibid,* #14.
[7]*Ibid,* #15–17.
[8]Ashley and O'Rourke, *op. cit.,*p. 5.

fidelity, and interpersonal presence. Although he used the term "soul," he was writing of the same embodied intelligent freedom as Fathers Ashley and O'Rourke. He wrote:

> The soul which is at the disposal of others is consecrated and inwardly dedicated; it is protected against suicide and despair, which are interrelated and alike, because it knows that it is not its own, and that the most legitimate use it can make of its freedom is precisely to recognize that it does not belong to itself.[9]

Marcel consciously used the term "mystery" to designate the human person and the experiences of the person like love and hope. *In a paradoxical sense, a major effort of Christian philosophy has been to recover the mystery of the person.* That mystery had been overlooked by trends in philosophy which reduced human persons to streams of consciousness or agents of conditioned reflex. In Marcel's view, persons enter an experience of mystery in their relationships with other persons, including the Person Who is God. Human community becomes a shared mystery.

Persons and Community

In fact, human persons cannot exist apart from human community. Every person has parents, and cannot develop either physically or psychologically without constant interpersonal relationships. Persons enrich themselves through language and learning, yet language presumes social relationships and persons who communicate with each other.

Among all God's creatures, only persons can appreciate the goodness of one another and love each other. *Love creates community and is the proper perfection of the person. To love another person and to allow oneself to be loved opens up degrees of knowledge otherwise unattainable.*

Yet life in community presents problems. Different groups may wish to structure community differently depending on their understanding of personal fulfillment. Pluralism means a variety of approaches, even to the basic notion of personal dignity and rights. Thus, some views of society would allow individual persons only to have full rights and dignity upon reaching a certain level of participation in society. Other

---

[9] Marcel, Gabriel, *The Philosophy of Existentialism* (New York, N.Y.: The Citadel Press, 1961), p. 43.

views would base personal rights on social contract theories or views in which individuals have no obligations to the community beyond their own selfish interests.

The vision of the person found in the Christian tradition of philosophy and developed in Biblical and theological reflection can serve as a leaven or yeast in a pluralistic society. All the many philosophies of the person and society grow out of common human experience and have major points of agreement.

A document like the United Nations' *Universal Declaration of Human Rights* represents an ethical consensus of the world's major religions, supposedly supported as well by Marxism and secular humanism. Two of its introductory articles represent a basic charter of the dignity of the human person:

> Article 1: *All human beings are born free and equal in dignity and rights. They are endowed with reason and conscience and should act toward one another in a spirit of brotherhood.*

> Article 3: *Everyone has the right to life, liberty and security of person.*[10]

Conclusion

This *Handbook on Critical Life Issues* has begun with a study of the person through reason and reflection *to provide a background for everything which follows.* The next chapter will provide a Biblical study of the person as a complement to this chapter. The other chapters of Part I will add to the study of the person in the Judeo-Christian tradition and Catholic teaching.

Part II will focus on the beginning of personhood and the related ethical issue of abortion. Part III will look at the responsibilities and rights of sick and suffering persons. It will include chapters on organ transplantation and determining when a person has truly died. Chapters 12 through 16 will examine ethical and legal aspects of decisions about taking life, allowing death, and prolonging life.

Admittedly, the brief chapters of this book offer only short discussions of specific critical issues in the life and death of human persons. The broader issues of world poverty, economic exploitation, and the insanity of the nuclear arms race are left aside completely.

---

[10]Cf. Ashley and O'Rourke, *op. cit.*, pp. 14–16.

Yet the specific issues presented here are in the context of the present commitment in the United States today to a pro-life ideology. Chapter 5 will present data gathered by Raymond Adamek showing the expansion of a pro-death ideology in the United States today. *Such an ideology does not enhance the mystery and dignity of the person. Nor does it offer much optimism for a hopeful approach to the broader social issues of poverty, exploitation, and the nuclear arms race.*

Discussion Questions

1. Why is the ability to "humanize" one's life a distinguishing characteristic of human persons?
2. Why can't human behavior be predicted by measuring the strength of personality traits?
3. What could you say to Aristotle to improve upon his definition of persons as "rational animals?"
4. How can freedom be considered the key to understanding the human person?
5. Why has a major effort of Christian philosophy been to recover the mystery of the person?
6. Can you suggest why some predominantly subjective views of the person provide a weak basis for the articles cited from the United Nations' Universal Declaration of Human Rights?

Preview of Chapter 2

• The Bible teaches primarily, not *what* the human person is, but *for Whom* the human person is: for God.

• The human person is called to a special relationship of intimacy with God.

• The human person is not equal to God, but is equal with all other human beings.

• The human person is a living body, not an incarnated soul.

• The human person is responsible for his or her actions.

• Christ is the New Person for the sake of new persons.

• The secret of being a person is to be loved and to love.

• Our being loved and our call to love is in the Sacrifice of Christ.

CHAPTER 2

The Person as Known in the Bible and Faith

Our understanding of what it means to be a human person has not remained static, but has grown with the growth of the revelation which is represented in the Bible and in the Faith of the Church. *Current understanding of the nature of man has evolved beyond that to be found in the Old and New Testaments or even in the earliest teachings of the Church.*

This should not surprise us, for even in the Scripture itself there is at least a hint that more could be said of the human person than the Bible actually says. Thus, for at least a few pages in the Book of Wisdom (2:22 and 3:4), Greek forms of thought are used to express trust in God for victory over death. More significantly, Genesis 1 seems to represent a somewhat more thoughtful view of the human person than the older view recorded in Genesis 2.

It is clear that the Bible writers intended to say the most important things about the human person for the sake of his or her relationship with God. All other subsequent attempts to understand the human person would have to be evaluated in the light of that relationship. Such attempts would include those of the Greeks to understand the mysterious power they called "the soul." They would include also the theories of present day psychiatry, sociology, physiology and philosophy.

The Bible does not attempt to give a scientific account of the working of the organs of the human body or to pursue questions concerning the existence of a non-material part of the human person that would account for human activities such as intellectual activity or free will. Whatever facts may be usefully noted about the human person in order to focus on his or her relationship to God are given and, indeed, insisted upon. There is in the Bible, however, no effort carefully to define terms so as to avoid all confusion. Still less is there any search for some consistent, underlying explanations as to *how* it is possible for the human person to think, feel, and the like.

Centuries after the Bible was completed, the Church found herself in a civilization that prized systematic, orderly thinking in science and philosophy. *It became important, and still is, for the Church to show how the teachings of the Bible concerning the nature of man are not inconsistent with new methods of thought, if they are used properly.*

The Bible: The Human Person Concentrating on God

The Bible says a great deal about the human person, but it concentrates on God and on getting the human person to concentrate on God. It does not attempt to study the human person for the sake of studying what makes up a human being, but for the sake of showing what makes up the human person's relationship to God. For instance, the Bible is not interested in what this or that part of the human person is (e.g., the heart or the hand), but how this or that part is *related to God.* It is not concerned with the part by itself, but rather the way that part represents the *whole person.* Thus, the "lifting up of the hands" in prayer is important only because the hands stand for the *whole person* lifting himself or herself up to God.

The Human Person: Meant for Other Persons

Exactly how this *whole person* is made up is simply not a concern of the Bible writers. What is their concern is that the human person is made for *other persons,* and primarily for the *Person Who is his Maker.*

Thus the emphasis is not on what the human person is, but on how the human person *came to be* and *continues to be*—namely, out of a relationship with the Lord. The Bible is not concerned with my exact nature as a person, but rather with the sustaining hand of God as He keeps me in existence. It does not pose questions about the existence of something called a soul, which might be the internal source of my bodily life. Instead, it explores the way in which a source outside of me keeps me living. The interest here is in the Lord God.

Thus in the Bible my *individuality* as a person is not treated as depending on my having a body which is distinct from everyone else's, but on my having to answer personally to the Lord for what I do. This does not deny that my physical or spiritual make-up may in some true sense make me an individual. The Bible is simply not concerned with that question. The only value in man which it treats is the value he has because his life and existence are a gift from God.

Not What You *Are*, But How You *Live With* God

The Bible states that the human person is made "in the image and likeness of God." (Gn. 1:26–27) That may or may not tell us of something which my body and my activities of thought and action *are*. The Bible, however, is here more concerned with what that tells us about what each of us is to *do*: (1) We are to enjoy an intense friendship with God which the other creatures do not; (2) We are to bring them into submission because we are special governors of God's creation. Without this friendship and collaboration with God, I will experience painfully just how unimportant I am, left to myself.

> All mankind is grass and all their glory like the flower of the field. The grass withers, the flower wilts, when the breath of the Lord blows upon it. So then, the people is the grass. (Is. 40:6–7)

Human Persons: Made for Human Persons

The necessity for a genuine relationship with God is mirrored in the human person's need for a genuine relationship with other human beings. The human person is most himself or herself when he or she is in relationship with others. The conjugal relationship is the model of this:

> The Lord God said: It is not good for the man to be alone. I will make a suitable partner for him. (Gn. 2:18)

The human person fulfills his or her relationship to God precisely by being in relationship with others:

> God created man in his image; in the divine image he created him; male and female he created them. (Gn. 1:27)

No earthly creature can be a true companion to me except another human being.

The Human Person is Special Only Because of God

Whatever is special about the human person comes from his or her having a relationship with God. This is a relationship which only God can establish, and He does so by doing something for human beings which He did not do for His other living creatures: God, in a special act, *breathes* into each person "the breath of life." (Gn. 27) Moreover, even the human physical structure is special because God carefully and devotedly "*formed*" the human person, whereas, the Bible account records, He only "*made*" the trees. (Gn. 2:8–9)

Then human beings enter into the governance of all things in the "garden" of creation. The reason the Bible gives for this honor is, not that human beings are so splendid, but simply that the Lord God chose to place human beings in this relationship of power over all things. He shares with them moreover, the wondrous and even divine power of speech by which they name the birds and animals and thus show themselves God's representatives.

> So the Lord God formed out of the ground various wild animals and various birds of the air, and he brought them to the man to see what he would call them; whatever the man called each of them would be its name. The man gave names to all the cattle, all the birds of the air, and all the wild animals. . . (Gn. 2:19–20)

Even work itself is a dignity which God bestows on the human person so that he or she may subdue the world which God has begun:

> Be fertile and multiply; fill the earth and subdue it. (Gn. 128)

Psalm 8 sums up what the human person's relationship to God has meant in a hymn of praise:

What is man that you should be mindful of him,
    or the son of man that you should care for him?
You have made him little less than the angels,
    and crowned him with glory and honor.
You have given him rule over the works of your hands,
    putting all things under his feet:
All sheep and oxen,
    yes, and the beasts of the field,
The birds of the air, the fishes of the sea,
    and whatever swims the paths of the sea,
O Lord, our Lord,
    how glorious is your name over all the earth! (Ps. 8:5–10)

Note that the psalm here makes no explicit mention of anything which is part of the human person and would make him or her fit for such royal power over the universe. If there is some such thing in the human person the Scriptures are silent on the matter. They are concerned not with what is *in the human person* but what is *in the relationship* which God has freely and lovingly bestowed upon that person.

The Human Person, God's Friend, But Never His Equal

Yet this very relationship of special closeness to the Lord God also brings out the distance between the human persons and their Maker. The human person receives; only God gives. It is the human person's to obey; God's to command.

> The Lord God gave man this order: 'You are free to eat from any of the trees of the garden except the tree of knowledge of good and bad. From that tree you shall not eat; the moment you eat from it you are surely doomed to die.' (Gn. 2:16–17)

Others Are Our Equals

This relationship with God is intimately bound up with the relationship to other human persons. Indeed, where the relationship with others is broken, the relationship with the Lord also is broken.

> You shall not bear hatred for your brother in your heart. Though you may have to reprove your fellow man, do not

incur sin because of him. Take no revenge and cherish no grudge against your fellow countrymen. You shall love your neighbor as yourself. (Lev. 19:17–18. See also versus 9–16)

Other persons are thus our equals not only in frailty and powerlessness before God, but also in their rights and dignity. It is interesting to note that the Bible never seeks to make the point that sin destroys the image of God which is in each of us.

The Human Person: A Life-Filled Body

But what has gone into the make-up of this creature upon whom God has bestowed so much? What *is* the human person? What *kind* of being is the human person?

The Scriptures are clear on one thing: The human person is a *body*. There is no thought of the human beings existing without existing as a body. The person is formed "of the clay of the ground" (Gn. 27) and, up until the moment that he is formed this way, there is no human being.

The Bible recognizes that this body to which life has been given is a unified whole, and not just a collection of assembled parts. It does not, however, make any effort to understand accurately and scientifically the nature of those parts, their inner workings, or their interconnections. The Bible is not concerned, for example, about the true physiological functioning of the brain and nervous system. It simply goes along with the general assumption of that day that the heart, not the brain and nervous system, is the "location" of our mind, our conscience, our knowledge, and of the free-will decisions which control our bodily movements.

The Human Person is Not a Spirit Which has Become "Incarnated"

Does the Bible indicate that the human person has a soul, i.e., a source within himself which makes the person's total being alive? The answer is: Yes! This soul is not, however, seen in the Old Testament as something which can continue to exist once the body has died. Indeed, when the Bible speaks of "the soul," it usually means the *whole person*, as is often the case when it speaks of "the hands," "the heart," or "the liver." *There is no doctrine in the Bible of a soul which in any way pre-exists the formation of the human body in which it becomes "incarnated."*

There is in the Old Testament—with the possible exception of the Book of Wisdom (2:22 and 34) not even any doctrine that a person can, as a soul, somehow survive death and live in "perfect happiness in heaven" without the body. Indeed it never occurs to the typical Old Testament writer to treat the human person as anything but a body-soul living being. Even when some effort is made to portray a kind of existence for the dead, it is a shadowy, feeble, and vague existence hardly able to be called life. To the king of Babylon who must face death, Isaiah says:

> The nether world below is all astir preparing for your coming; it awakens the shades to greet you, all the leaders of the earth . . . You too have become weak like us; you are the same as we . . . The couch beneath you is the maggot, your covering, the worm. (Is. 149–11)

Not exactly a picture of bliss!

The Human Person and His Personal Response

The human person is not merely an image of God, but a *living* image. The Bible pictures a whole array of the sentiments and emotions the human person experiences. More important, the human person is one to whom God can and does give authority, and from whom God expects a free and responsible use of that authority. The human person is capable of *understanding* what God requires of him or her, and of *freely choosing* to comply. He also refuses compliance, of course; indeed his life is a history of rebellions.

> For I acknowledge my offense and my sin is before me always. (Ps. 515)

Sin as the source of misery is not part of the Bible's definition of man. The human person is not made of evil (as some of the ancient pagan myths would have it), for the person is capable of following God in faith, which brings the guarantee of joy.

> Why are you so downcast, O my soul?
>   Why do you sigh within me?
> Hope in God! For I shall again be thanking him,
>   in the presence of my saviour and my God.
> (Ps. 43:5)

From the very beginning, then, in the Genesis story itself, the human person freely chooses a response to the special relationship God is offering to His creature. Whatever evil and anxiety the human person knows is traceable to a deliberate lack of faith in God and His offer.

"What is Man That You Should Be Mindful of Him, O Lord?"

The Bible, then, gives a portrait of human persons in all their nobility of body, joys and sorrows, guilt and innocence, fears and serenity, understanding and ignorance, freedom and enslavements, loving and rebellious responses to God.

Why does the Bible note all this? Not out of a primary concern to analyze the human person, but because all of these elements of human life are part of a relationship which God wishes the human person to have, a covenant or bond which God wishes to share with the human person. The full nature of this bond was to be revealed only with appearance of Jesus in Israel's last days. The New Testament is concerned with unfolding what the Christ shows to each human being about what it means to be a person. *Indeed, Jesus makes it possible for each of us not only to know what it is to be a new person but actually to be one.*

The New Adam and the New Person

Jesus sees the human person as we have seen that person pictured in the Jewish Scriptures. An important change, however, is Jesus' call to face courageously our limitations, fears, and sinfulness, and His offer of a change in ourselves, from the very roots of our being up. The choice must be made: continue in sin, or become, through Him, a new person. Fundamental to our acceptance of Him as the one and only Savior is our recognition of all others as equal to us and called with us to be new persons. Jesus is here to draw us to the truth about what, through desires created and kept alive in our hearts by God, we want to be.

"I am the way, and the truth, and the life." (Jn. 14:6) And what is this truth which Jesus is? Certainly it is the truth about the Father and His unique relationship to Jesus Himself. But why is Jesus revealing *this*? He does it that we might become truly *living persons:*

> If you live according to my teaching, you are truly my disciples; then you will know the truth, and the truth will set you free. (Jn. 8:31–32)

21

The Secret of Being a Person

In revealing Himself as the restorer of our freedom to respond worthily to God, what does Jesus reveal to us? He reveals His *love*. And what does His love reveal to us? It reveals the love of the *Father*. Jesus and His Father are persons only because they are in a communion of love "projected to infinity," to the point, Christian theologians would later sense, that their Love Itself is a Person—the Spirit.

This means that one cannot be a person without being called to be in a communion of love with others. The more truly we love, the more intensely we become persons. Love alone enables the Father, the Son, and the Holy Spirit to be Individuals, and yet a perfect Unity. And love alone enables us to be *persons,* to be individuals who are nonetheless united with God and among ourselves. Even more fundamentally, love alone enables us to be at one with the one God Who is three Persons.

"Redeemer of Man"

This love which is the life possessed by the Father, the Son and the Holy Spirit is revealed, not just as God's life, but as His life offered to us. It is offered to us in the condition in which we find ourselves, in all our misery and sinfulness. Without this love's being revealed and offered to us, we would not know what love is. In other words, we would be less and less *persons.*

> The way we came to understand love was that he laid down his life for us. (1 Jn. 3:16)

> God's love was revealed in our midst in this way: he sent his only Son to the world that we might have life through him. Love then consists in this: not that we have loved God, but that He has loved us and sent his Son as an offering for our sins. (1 Jn. 4:9–10)

What it means to be a person, then, is revealed in the life which exists among the three Persons Who are the One God: a life of perfect communion in love. This love in God is revealed to human beings and offered for their sharing. In that revelation and offer, the human person comes to understand what it is to *be* a person and is enabled to become *more* a person. This revelation and offer is made to the human person specifically in the events of Holy Week called "the Paschal Mystery": the Death and Resurrection of the Lord Jesus.

It is in this Paschal Mystery that we find out what it means for God to be three Persons, and what it means for us to be persons by sharing in their life. In other words, we find out what love is. Pope John Paul II writes in his inaugural encyclical:

> Man cannot live without love. He remains a being that is incomprehensible for himself, *his life is senseless, if love is not revealed to him, if he does not encounter love, if he does not experience love and make it his own, if he does not participate intimately in it.* This, as has already been said, is why Christ the Redeemer "fully reveals man to himself." This is the *human dimension* of the mystery of the Redemption." (That is, it reveals who man is.) In this dimension man finds again the greatness, dignity and value that belong to his humanity.[1] (emphasis added)

Later the Pope cites the Second Vatican Council:

> By his Incarnation he, the son of God, in a certain way united himself to each person.[2]

The Holy Father then continues:

> Each one is included in the mystery of the Redemption and with each one Christ has united himself forever through this mystery. Every man . . . *each one* of the four-thousand million human beings living on our planet has become a sharer (in Jesus Christ) from the moment he is conceived beneath the heart of his mother.[3]

To be a person means to be the object of divine love and to be called to live in that communion of love.

Discussion Questions

1. Did the Bible writers intend to give us all possible details, including scientific ones, about what it means to be human, or do they limit themselves to only certain aspects?

---

[1]Pope John Paul II, *The Redeemer of Man (Redemptor Hominis)*. (Boston, MA: Daughters of St. Paul Press, 1979), # 10, p. 18.
[2]*The Church in the Modern World (Gaudium et Spes)*, #22.
[3]Pope John Paul II, *op. cit.*, # 13, pp. 25–26.

2. What passage in the book of Genesis points to the fact that the human person needs other human persons?
3. What are the indications in the Book of Genesis that the human person has a relationship with God which the other creatures do not have?
4. The Book of Wisdom, written close to the birth of Christ, teaches clearly that there is a real and joyous life after death for the human being who is faithful to God. Was this always clear to the Bible writers in the centuries before the Book of Wisdom?
5. What are some of the promises of Jesus for making us fully human?

Preview of Chapter 3

• The fact that adequate health care must meet the spiritual psychological, and physiological needs of the person indicates the richness and complexity of being a person.

• Research has proven clear connections between the *psyche* (mind or soul) and the *soma* (body). Psychosomatic medicine treats physical ailments produced by anxiety and its emotional derivatives.

• Human persons are health stewards. Optimal human functioning on all levels of the personality produces health.

• Holistic medicine programs include all levels of human need and are often church-related.

• One's faith-filled "outlook on life" and spiritual well-being can foster physical health, hence the Church has a special role in health ministry.

CHAPTER 3

Person-Centered Health Care

"The Catholic health care facility recognizes *the spiritual, psychological, and physiological needs of the person.*" This statement expresses the theme of this chapter. It comes from a publication of the Catholic Health Association which presents criteria for self-evaluation by Catholic health care facilities.[1]

This volume on critical life issues includes these first three chapters about the human person as essential preparation for a satisfactory discussion of the ethical issues affecting life and health. For instance, this chapter will argue that the human person can never receive adequate health care without recognition of the three kinds of needs mentioned above.

If, then, the actual provision of adequate health care necessarily includes the spiritual, psychological, and physiological needs of the per-

---

[1]*Evaluative Criteria for Catholic Health Care Facilities* (St. Louis, MO, Catholic Health Association, 1980), p. 21.

son, *a statement has been made about the definition of a person.* In other words, the necessarily complex character of health care demonstrates the richness and complexity of being a person.

But this richness and complexity, in turn, add depth and ethical significance to the inviolability of the life of an innocent person. (Chapter 4) It also influences all the discussions of abortion, suicide, euthanasia, organ transplants, prolonging life decisions, and determination of death to be found in this book.

Hence, the first part of this chapter will discuss "Medicine and the Person" to present an overview of the interaction of body, mind, and spirit in the person who receives health care. *The contemporary interest in preventative health care also reveals the intimate connection between bodily health and mental attitudes.* This will be discussed under the heading "Stewardship of Health." Finally, the chapter will conclude with practical information about holistic health programs which integrate the spiritual, psychological, and physiological care of human persons.

Medicine and the Person

Medical schools today communicate to future physicians a vast amount of information about the human body, both its organic structure and its biochemical processes. Basic medicine divides its study of the human body into the nine organ systems, each of which has organs with specific functions.

The nervous system, with the intimately related endocrine system, coordinates the other seven organ systems which are related in a complex manner. Of the other seven systems, the reproductive system has special importance. It is involved in the continuity of the human species and it offers the individual the opportunity of founding a family community.

The other six organ systems of the human body are the skeletal and muscular, integumentary (skin), alimentary (stomach and digestion), respiratory, circulatory, and excretory (bodily waste) systems.

Modern medicine has accumulated a phenomenal knowledge of all nine organ systems, their proper functioning, and their misfunctioning. Physicians can often use extremely sophisticated diagnostic equipment to uncover maladies in any of them, and any abnormality whatever of the human body.

But modern medicine has come to realize more and more clearly that one can give health care only to persons, not to bodies. Psychosomatic medicine has proven amazing relationships between bodily ailments and the mental or emotional disposition of persons. The term "psychosomatic" comes

27

from the Greek *psyche* (mind or soul) and *soma* (body). Some psychiatrists object to using the term because it may imply a separation of these two elements of the human person or a simple relationship between them—as if each would mirror the other.

The term "psychosomatic medicine" came into common usage in the 1930s as research showed more and more instances of mind-body interaction. A special journal, *Psychosomatic Medicine,* was launched in 1939. Research has demonstrated the role of psychological stress in the origin of such physical conditions as hypertension (high blood pressure), peptic ulcers, bronchial asthma, coronary heart disease, migraine headaches, diabetes, diarrhea, skin acne, constipation, and gout.

Research further indicates that anxiety and its emotional derivatives play a key role in producing such ailments. The anxiety may even remain unconscious for the most part, and still the physiological repercussions occur. Bodily reactions that accompany emotional states indicate the close interplay of body and mind. Fear or anger, as emotions, stimulate protective and defensive reactions of the body. Physical ailments usually arise when emotions are not discharged properly, as when they are an unconscious response to a stressful situation.

Among the more unusual examples of psychosomatic neurotic reactions are instances of "conversion hysteria." In this situation tensions generated on the level of psychological experience produce disturbances in a person's sensory or muscular abilities so they cannot see or hear or walk. Yet the physical apparatus for these functions remains intact. One can notice readily that such cases lend themselves to rather miraculous healing!

The muscle system of the human body can also respond to emotional anxiety with various kinds of spasms. Continuous misuse of the muscles for expressing anxiety has a tiring effect, giving rise to certain types of backache, even rheumatic pains.

The branch of medicine which specializes in disorders of the *psyche* (mind or soul) is psychiatry. This discipline proceeds from a basis in general medical knowledge to specialized knowledge of mental disorders. The fact that contemporary psychiatry can successfully relieve many forms of mental illness by prescribing medication indicates the close interworking of *soma* (body) and *psyche.*

Psychiatry has come into its own in the 20th century with tremendous advances in the diagnosis and cure of mental illness. Sigmund Freud opened new frontiers with his analysis of the unconscious. Yet Hippocrates, in the fourth century before Christ, invoked physiological theories to explain instances of mental derangement. For instance, he discussed the causative role of yellow and black bile in mental disorders. He also catalogued various syndromes of mental illness with descriptions that are still useful.

Modern medicine deals with the mental and emotional life of persons through tranquilizers and other mood-altering drugs. These medications can allay anxieties and even eliminate hallucinations. The physicians who prescribe them wield tremendous power over the personality and behavior of their patients. Proper use of all these drugs requires great knowledge, training, and skill.

Narcotic drugs such as opium, morphine, heroin, codeine, marijuana, and cocaine, all exert an extraordinary influence over the mental and emotional states of persons using them. Drug addiction leads to moral degradation by the enslaving of human freedom. The effect of drugs on the mind and behavior offers another instance of body/mind interaction.

This discussion of "body medicine" and "mind medicine" has illustrated a basic and important theme. The theme is simply this: *Modern medicine proves the mysterious complexity of the human person by the numerous avenues it uses to approach both bodily and mental health, and by its research on the interrelation of the two.*

Stewardship of Health

In California, pet owners can enroll their dogs or cats in an animal version of Blue Cross for animal health care. The annual premium varies, according to the age and breed of the pet, from as little as $20 to over a $100. The veterinarians who have sponsored the program would undoubtedly prefer it if the pets stayed healthy. The fewer the visits to the animal hospital, the more profitable the plan for those who administer it.

Yet cats and dogs do not really take responsibility for their own health. Nature has given them certain instincts telling them to avoid moving automobiles and electric fences. But, if they cuddle in a dog blanket or wear a collar which reflects in the dark, it is the foresight of their human master which provided this.

Human persons not only protect the health of their pets; first and foremost, they act as stewards of their own health. The health of cats and dogs may be affected by air pollution, but the pets have no way of correcting this. Human persons assume responsibility for protecting their health and, in a democratic society, they participate in the public efforts to overcome pollution and create a healthy environment.

This emphasizes another facet of the difference between human persons and other living creatures. Only persons are health stewards. The health or disease of pets and other animals does not depend on their attitudes, values, or life choices. But the attitudes, values, and life choices of human beings determine, to a very large extent, their state of health.

29

What is human health? The World Health Organization in 1958 declared: "Health is a state of complete physical, mental, and social well-being, and not merely the absence of disease or infirmity."[2] This rather vague description has, at least, the advantage of emphasizing the positive aspects of health in the reference to "physical, mental, and social well-being."

Fathers Ashley and O'Rourke in their masterful volume, *Health Care Ethics,* have reviewed much modern literature that describes human health. They propose a variation on the World Health Organization description in terms of the four interrelated levels of human needs: *Human health is the optimal functioning of the human organism to meet biological, psychological, ethical, and spiritual needs."*[3]

This description indicates that human health will be impaired when human needs are left unfulfilled on any of the four levels. It suggests that biological health cannot be maintained in the face of a person's psychological, ethical, or spiritual "sickness."

The review of psychosomatic medicine already presented in this chapter supports this broad notion of human health. The tension and anxiety which lead to biological illness originate when a person's psychological, ethical, or spiritual needs are not met.

The recent widespread interest of many Americans in jogging as a form of exercise illustrates this. Persons who jog are not only exercising bodily muscles, they are withdrawing from the pressures of daily duties for periods of solitude and reflection. Joggers relax their minds and even commune with God while trotting along the highway or path. No wonder jogging is considered "healthy."

A prominent example of physical illness that may have originated from the other levels of the human personality could be former President Nixon's bout with thrombophlebitis, the development of blood clots in his leg, during the Watergate scandal. The enormous stress he experienced must have been psychological, ethical, and spiritual in origin.

Since human health derives from optimal human functioning on all four levels of the human person, a great variety of professional persons can contribute to human health. Physicians and psychologists specialize in biological and psychological aspects of health. But many other persons, including clergy and wise counselors, help people provide for their spiritual and ethical needs and health.

---

[2] See discussion article by Callahan, Daniel, "The WHO Definition of Health," *Hastings Center Studies.* 1, no. 3:77–87.

[3] Ashley, O.P., Benedict M. and O'Rourke, O.P., Kevin D., *Health Care Ethics,* A Theological Analysis (St. Louis MO, Catholic Health Association, 2nd Edit., 1982), pp. 21–37, especially p. 26.

Self-Care

In this sense, every person "doctors" himself or herself. One of the best-known experts on self-help in health care and preventative medicine for adults, Dr. James F. Fries, has become the same kind of oracle as Dr. Benjamin Spock became in the field of child care. His book, co-authored with Donald M. Vickery M.D., is entitled *Take Care of Yourself— A Consumer's Guide to Medical Care*.[4] It has sold 1 1/2 million copies.

Dr. Fries points out that people go to the doctor only about 20% of the times when they feel sick. The rest of the time they buy over-the-counter medications and doctor themselves. If only 2% of the people who buy such medicine actually went to physicians, it would increase by 62% the number of doctor-visits and the number of doctors needed for the United States population.[5]

Wellness programs to assist people with their own health care have sprung up all over the United States. Often business corporations support or encourage such programs for the sake of business efficiency. Dr. Fries cites one company which found that work-days lost per employee per year dropped from 6.2 days to 4.8 days because of his program of self-care.

Hospitals are becoming more and more conscious of the possibilities of assisting people to foster their own health. Many hospitals have actually changed their legal names to become "health centers."

Providence Hospital in Cincinnati, OH, opened a Health Awareness Program on Sept. 1, 1979.[6] Dr. Thomas Spasoff, P.Ed.D., the director, describes health awareness as an ongoing process, initiated by the individual, leading toward a better relationship between the mind, body, spirit and emotions. The major components of his program include nutritional guidance, physical conditioning, stress management, environmental appreciation, medical self-care, and smoking cessation. Dr. Spasoff speaks on health awareness to religious and civic groups several times weekly. He has supervised health awareness days at major shopping malls and appears frequently on television.

These efforts at health awareness and disease prevention dramatize the theme of stewardship of health. Human persons experience health as something complex and profound unlike that of the domestic animals covered by the health care program in California. *This serves to reinforce the central claim in this volume that human persons enjoy a kind of existence which is unparalleled in the world of creation.* The Church teaches the inher-

---

[4]Reading, MA: Addison-Wesley Publishers, 1981.

[5]Harris, T. George, "Conversation: Dr. James Fries," *American Health*, July/August, 1982, pp. 42–47, at p. 45.

[6]"Profile," *Hospital Progress*, Ap. 1982, p. 34.

ent dignity, rights, and responsibilities of persons. It also has a ministry of health in the tradition of Jesus, the divine Healer.

The Church and Holistic Health

Dr. Granger E. Westberg, D.D., is a Lutheran clergyman who is the founder and president emeritus of Wholistic Health Centers, Inc., with headquarters in Hinsdale, Illinois, near Chicago. Wholistic Health Centers are medical clinics conducted in hospitals, churches, and colleges where the physicians and nurses are assisted by clergy who are trained as counselors to deal with the spiritual dimensions of illness. *In these Centers the staff uses an interdisciplinary approach to health care, dealing especially with problems of the human spirit.*

Dr. Richard H. Lange wrote about Granger Westberg's work in the *New York State Journal of Medicine:*

> The distinguishing factor of these centers is the practice of scientific medicine with all patients receiving a full medical work-up to uncover any organic diseases. In addition, health education and preventive medicine are emphasized since holistic doctrine implies individual responsibility and activated patients . . . These preventive measures and common sense approaches can be an effective complement to today's highly technologic and highly specialized medicine and should be welcomed as old friends. They may need fresh introduction to some of our more technologic and narrowly focused colleagues, but they are nevertheless part of the tradition of medicine.[7]

Wholistic Health Centers can be located in churches as part of its health ministry, and sometimes are. But since this is not often feasible, what other alternatives are there?

Dr. Westberg's daughter, Jill, is working with several churches to develop a health ministry. At her congregation of the Lutheran Church in America a "Health Cabinet" has been formed. Most homes have a medicine cabinet, so this church now has a health cabinet. *The Health Cabinet is actually a group of volunteers who are concerned about health and committed to seeing that the congregation carries on a healing ministry.*

The Health Cabinet assists individuals and families to become increasingly responsible for maintaining and improving their own health

---

[7]Lange, Dr. Richard H., "Wholistic Medicine: Is All Wholistic Medicine Whole?" *N.Y. State Journal of Medicine.* May, 1980, Vol. 80, No. 6, pp. 996–99.

and that of their community. The Cabinet is not involved in diagnosis and treatment. This is the domain of the person's family physician. The Health Cabinet seeks to act as a strong influence in the life of the congregation to ensure that the stewardship of health is expressed in worship, education, networks of support, and recreation.

The Health Cabinet works in three main areas. *The first is through sponsoring health-related changes or activities through already existing "structures" such as the worship, religious education classes, and youth groups.* For instance, a member of the Health Cabinet might offer to teach a session in various religious education classes for different ages on "Your Faith and Your Health." Or, at a social event that is scheduled by another organization, people may be encouraged to bring to the potluck "healthy-type" foods to share the experience of eating healthy food that is also tasty.

A second front in which the Health Cabinet involves itself is the sponsorship of new programs or activities without going through already existing structures. The Health Cabinet might put on a "Health Fair" that devotes a particular Sunday to the healing ministry. This includes a worship service as well as activities after the service—a sermon on the healing elements of faith, contemporary readings on how faith is actually related to health, and Biblical readings which refer to the healings of Jesus. After the service, there may be activities that involve people in various stress testing exercises. These activities could be followed by a potluck lunch of healthy foods which are described, with recipes provided, by the persons who brought them.

A third area of activity is a survey of the overall health and unhealth in the life of the whole congregation. This leads to efforts at supporting health in a collective way. It means developing a network of resources within the community, the resources being the people and what they have to offer to one another. This kind of mutual assistance reaches out to persons who are suffering psychologically and spiritually, as well as physically.

This kind of Health Cabinet leadership described by Jill Westberg could easily be adopted in Catholic parishes. In the parish organizational structure that has developed since the Second Vatican Council many parishes have commissions on ecumenism, social justice, and education. *Why not a Commission on Health and Healing?*

Dr. Granger Westberg cites a four-decade study of the health of Harvard graduates which shows that mental and emotional stress always precedes physical illness.[8] He sees as an essential remedy for such stress

---

[8]Vaillant, George E., "Natural History of Male Psychologic Health, Effects of Mental Health on Physical Health," *New England Journal of Medicine*. Dec. 6, 1979, Vol. 301, No. 23, pp. 1249–54.

an "outlook on life" which relates to one's faith, value system, and spiritual life.

Hence, the churches are very important in helping people stay healthy. In the early history of the United States the numerous Catholic hospitals were founded to meet grave needs in caring for the sick, especially the sick who were poor. *In this last part of the 20th century, the Church seems called to broaden its health ministry toward stimulating health awareness and person-centered health care.*

Conclusion

This chapter has viewed health care in the context of the spiritual and psychological, as well as physiological, needs of human persons. The need for, and success of, person-centered health care gives proof of the unique meaning and dignity of human personhood. The next chapter will explore the ethical norm of the inviolability of the lives of innocent human persons.

Discussion Questions

1. Give examples of psychosomatic ailments affecting as many of the nine organ systems of the body as you can.
2. Give examples of other public figures, like former President Nixon, who has seemed to experience psychosomatic ailments.
3. What are some examples of helpful and wholesome psychosomatic interactions?
4. How would you separate the roles of psychiatry and religious counseling in health care?
5. What do you think of the definitions of human health given in this chapter?
6. Why does the Harvard study cited by Dr. Westberg indicate that the Church has a role in health care?

Preview of Chapter 4

- Each person is a living portrait of God Himself.

- The first pages of the Bible are a protest against any cheapening of our concept of the human person.

- The Human Person is more than a merely material animal because he can detect the intelligent free actions of others, and act with intelligent freedom himself.

- What we do to a person's body we do to the person himself.

- No one can destroy another person's right to live.

- One may at times allow the death of the innocent to occur, but may never aim at causing it.

CHAPTER 4

The Inviolability of Each Human Life

A key document of the Second Vatican Council of all the Bishops of the Catholic Church, held in Rome from 1962 to 1965, applies Catholic teaching and the Judeo-Christian heritage to the problems of the modern world. Its title is, "The Church in the Modern World."

In one optimistic sentence, that document presents the basic principle of Christian ethics: "There is a growing awareness of the sublime dignity of the human person, who stands above all things and whose rights and duties are universal and inviolable."[1]

Subsequently this document describes grave crimes which poison civilization, militate against the honor of the Creator, and debase those who commit them more than the victims. Heading the list are offenses against life itself, such as murder, genocide, abortion, euthanasia, and wilful suicide.[2]

---

[1]*The Church in the Modern World (Gaudium et Spes)*, # 26.
[2]*ibid.* # 27.

Later chapters of this *Handbook* discuss the practices of abortion, euthanasia, and suicide. But this chapter concerns the basic principle which they offend: the inviolability of innocent human life. Notice the word "innocent." Judeo-Christian ethics has protected human life without excluding killing in capital punishment and also has allowed for deaths resulting from just war or self-defense.

The core principle of inviolability as the Catholic Church upholds it says: *One may never aim to destroy the bodily life of an innocent person.* May one tolerate such destruction? Perhaps. May one question precisely when a new human life begins? Surely. May one wonder when death has actually occurred? Definitely. But may one aim to destroy innocent human life? NEVER!

The Human Person—A Living Portrait of His Maker

Why such a conviction on the part of the Church? Because God has given her the clear knowledge that *the human person's created in the image of God himself.* It is as simple as that. This fact of the human person's being in the image of God is basic to all Christian consideration of what one should or should not do to human life. The Church sees this belief as established by the Holy Spirit Himself in the faith of the chosen bearers of His benevolence in history. Thus, among the chosen people of the Old Testament, this fundamental conviction shows itself in the very opening pages of the Book of Genesis, where God is pictured as saying:

> "Let us make mankind in our image and likeness ... God created man in His image. In the image of God He created them." (Gn. 1:26–27).

While it is true that all life of any kind whatsoever comes from God, *human* life comes in a very special manner. God breathed the breath of life into the first human creature (Gn. 2:7), and without this gift no human creature would be alive (Jb. 34:14ff). Human blood represented human life in the Old Testament and belongs to God because the human person is His image. "If anyone sheds the blood of man, by man shall his blood be shed; for in the image of God has man been made." (Gn. 9:6)

A passage in Deuteronomy focuses on the necessity of expressing reverence for the sacredness of the life of a murder victim by always executing the murderer. (Dt. 21: 1–9). In this passage a detailed ritual tells the elders of the city nearest which a murder victim is found what to do when the murderer cannot be found and executed. For whether the criminal can be found or not, the sacredness of the spilt blood must be expressed: "Absolve, O Lord, your people Israel, whom you have ransomed, and let not the guilt of shedding innocent blood remain in the midst of your people Israel."

A respected Protestant scholar of the Old Testament summarized God's exclusive right to dominion over human life:

> All human life, with other forms of life also drawn in along the way, is tied to its Creator and Sustainer and Consummator in such a way that it is simply not the prerogative of any human being to dispose of such life except as the human being, or the community, can claim to be acting directly on behalf of God in doing so.[3]

The Bible: A Protest Against a Lower Estimate of The Human Person

The Bible's picture of man stands in stark contrast to pagan myths written in the same period as the Book of Genesis. In many of these myths—stories that show what pagans believed about their gods—the human person was *not* made in the image and likeness of the Living God. To the contrary: in one mythical story, for example, the world was made out of the cut up body of Tiamat, the most malevolent of the goddesses, and the human race from the butchered bones and compressed blood of Kingu, her evil consort.

The gods who were Tiamat's children rose up in rebellion against her and Kingu. Having done them in, Tiamat's children could think of nothing better "to do with the bodies" than to cut them up and make of them the world and a race of groveling slaves to serve them. And supposedly from this cruelty, hatred, and violence came forth—*the human race!* One of the main messages behind this myth, then, is that human beings are made of basically evil stuff, are beneath any esteem from their makers (the gods), and are certainly incapable of any kind of intimacy with them.

It was against such a gloomy evaluation of the human race and the persons who constitute it that the Holy Spirit moved the Israelites and their prophets to give us the Genesis portrait of the human person who is a portrait of the One Living God of all power, beauty, and love.

---

[3]Harrelson, Walter, *The Ten Commandments and Human Rights* (Philadelphia: Fortress Press, 1980), p. 119.

Let us make mankind in our image and likeness. Let them have dominion over the fish of the sea, the birds of the air, the cattle, over the wild animals, and every creature that crawls on earth . . . God created man in His image . . . In the image of God He created Him. (Gn. 1:26–27)

Whatever dignity all of these fish and birds and cattle and any other creatures had, it was totally transcended by the majesty of the *one* creature who had dominion over them all because this creature alone was in the image of God. Throughout the Old Testament, this vision of the human person shows itself again and again.

What is man that you should be mindful of him, or the son of man that you should care for him? You have made him little less than the angels and crowned him with glory and honor. You have given him rule over the works of your hands, putting all things under his feet. (Ps. 8:5–7)

For God formed man to be imperishable; the image of His own nature he made him. (Wis. 2:23)

It is not surprising then that the Church has this most basic of all convictions about the human person. We are made in the image of God. A society which is convinced it must carry on the practical matters of its day-to-day life as if God did not exist pays little attention to this conviction that the human person is made in the image of God. To hold this conviction and to express it is to "give witness" in the truest sense of that term, for this conviction represents a truth which the secularist mentality finds threatening.

Nonetheless, the dignity of the human person which comes from that person's being incomparably the image of God on this earth is so impressive that it cannot escape the notice of many non-Christians, and even of some who do not believe in God. This is not surprising, for this dignity of the human person can be obvious to purely human reason, even when left on its own. Moreover, as the Second Vatican Council teaches, even outside the visible communion of the church the Holy Spirit is not absent to the workings of the human mind. No wonder there are found men and women of good will who do not consciously share the Christian Faith in its entirety, but who do share at least some spiritual understanding of the unique dignity of each person.

This is why recent Popes have referred with hopefulness to the preamble of the United Nation's Universal Declaration of Human Rights. The language of this document was designed to bridge a gap between members of different religions, as well as between believers and non-believers. It speaks in terms of the "inherent dignity" and "inalienable rights" of each member of the human race. Hence conscientious people everywhere who want to see and respect the truth about the human person become allies in upholding the inviolability of innocent human life.

Still, the weight of witnessing to the human person's true worth falls especially upon the shoulders of those blessed with the Gospel and the teaching office of the Church and her bishop-shepherds. One truth to which the Catholic Church bears special witness today is, of course, that this dignity of the human person is found in a special way in the soul, the spiritual dimension of human nature. Yet this same dignity is also found in a definite, even though subordinate way in the body: its form, its organs, and its functioning. The body itself is, as the old Baltimore Catechism said, *in the image of God.*

The Human Person: A Body and More

Each person is in the image of God because he or she possesses this image in common with all human beings *universally*, that is, in the *same basic way*. The same imaging of God which is in *one* is in *all*. This is true of all human beings in their bodies, but especially in their souls. The soul of each person does not dwell in its human body like a tenant in an apartment, but its presence gives unified life to the "embodied person." The soul, together with its body, makes the human person mirror the glory of God as no other creature of God can possibly do.

The fish of the sea, the birds of the air, and all the other creatures do, of course, in some way mirror God.

> The heavens show forth the glory of God, and the earth proclaims His wonder. (Ps. 19:1)

Yet one rarely speaks of the "dignity" of non-human creatures; and then, it is usually because they bear some similarity to the human person. For only human beings, among all material creatures, have dignity, i.e., *worth* which is above that of merely material beings. Only human beings can know God's plan in the world He has made, for only human beings have an intellect; only human beings can freely follow that plan, for only human beings have a will. Only the human person can put a personal message and meaning into material things, from the soaring

40

spires of a cathedral built to God's honor to simple words of love to a spouse or a child. Only the human person can thus receive, share, and duplicate the creative intent and love of our Maker. This is the richness of existence universal to all human beings.

The autonomy and inviolability of every human person flows from this common sharing in the same dignity and destiny. Human persons can allow themselves to be sacrificed for the good of humanity, but not as if they were parts of a whole. For instance, if a person donates a kidney to someone, this is an act of charity, but not an interchanging of organs between two persons who are parts of one whole.

Pope Pius XII in 1956 rejected such a notion when considering the question of organ transplants. To take an organ from one person for the good of another *as if* both the persons and their organs were both subordinated to some larger whole would violate the rights of persons since persons are autonomous and inviolable.

Hence, the familiar principle of each individual's "right to life" should be rooted in the act of God which creates and sustains each human person. Christian theology understands that act as one which establishes and maintains the unique spiritual animation of the human body. Each human being represents a separate and autonomous individual.

What We Do to the Body, We Do to the Human Person.

The right to life—bodily life—is given to the human person by the Creator, not out of any whim of generosity, but out of God's own faithfulness to Himself and to His own decision in creating the human person in His image. God has created the human person as a *corporeal* creature. It is God's own decision that, *without a bodily nature*, the human person would not be the human person. For the Israelites, this fact of revelation (a fact detectable also by the natural power of reason, as many great minds have shown) meant that the human person needs a body in the same way a triangle needs three sides. Biblical writers do not see this inviolability as extending to every single individual, without exception. This is obvious in the case of capital punishment cited above, where, at least by God's extension of authority to the community, human life could indeed be taken.

The Church, however, has been forced to face the question of the inviolability of human life at another level: Are there *some* categories of persons whose life society never, under any circumstances, has authority from God to take? And if so, why? In this process of asking questions which Biblical writers did not focus upon, the "code word" of the Church's growing clarity of doctrine became: _Innocence._

Hence, capital punishment can be theoretically justified only on the supposition that a person _has lost a basic innocence_ by violating another human being made in the image and likeness of God, and that society _can know_ that the violation was a free, personal decision. This is the only basis which the Catholic Church has recognized as even possibly justifying capital punishment in a given case: That any criminal to be executed has, by a free personal act, destroyed the very right to live.

"The State," wrote Pius XII in 1952, "does not have at its disposal the individual's right to life. It . . . is allowed to the public authorities to deprive the condemned of the benefit of life . . . when already, by his crime, _he_ has himself destroyed _his own_ right to life."[4]

It seems that Pius XII here is simply recognizing the teaching of St. Thomas Aquinas, who, in discussing capital punishment, notes that the vicious criminal has, by a capital crime, "lost his human dignity in so far as that dignity means that he is a free man and exists in his own right. He lowers himself to the level of beasts, and like them is at the disposition of others for whatever is best for them."[5] Where a person has not, by a deliberate act, freely destroyed the very right to live, no one else can morally destroy it.

This doctrine, which allows killing those who are no longer innocent, remains controversial even despite the Old Testament precedent where God is thought of as ordering the taking of the life of murderers. Loss of innocence on which capital punishment is based cannot be easily established by human tribunals. Before civil society can correctly proceed it must establish the serious moral guilt of the criminal in a court of law. Human justice falls notoriously short of divine justice.

Furthermore, the three practical reasons usually advanced for the usefulness of capital punishment do not convince all civil and religious leaders today. Each of the reasons (retribution, deterrence, and reform) justify punishment, but not necessarily capital punishment. In fact, the United States Bishops in 1974 declared their opposition to capital punishment, and then, in November, 1980, published a pastoral statement supporting that opposition.[6]

It must be admitted, then, that there has been constant growth in the Church's perception of how this conviction of the inviolability of innocent human life is to be applied. And the growth continues. The

---

[4]Pius XII, "The Intangibility of the Human Person," Sept. 13, 1952, in _The Human Body_ (Boston: Daughters of St. Paul, 1969, pp. 205–206.

[5]_Summa Theologica, Secunda Secundae_, q. 64, a. 2.

[6]"Statement on Capital Punishment," _Origins_, Nov. 27, 1980, Vol. 10, No. 24.

present controversy over the problem of capital punishment is evidence that the Church does not always find such application easy.

The Church's Conviction Clarifies Itself ⇐

In addition to dealing with these issues as they arise from society's experiences, the Church is faced with puzzles arising from Biblical revelation as well. The Scriptures clearly record the conviction of some of the Patriarchs of Israel that God directly ordered them to take the lives of persons who were unquestionably innocent. For instance, God seemed to order Abraham to kill his innocent son, Isaac, as well as other people—women and infants included—in his wars with pagan tribes. St. Thomas Aquinas attempted to explain these orders by appealing to God's right to do anything He chooses.

Some present-day theologians question the adequacy of this explanation, seeing in it a hint that God can be self-contradictory and therefore unfaithful to Himself. They fear that this implies a view called "voluntarism" in which God determined morality purely by an act of divine will. Be that as it may, contemporary Bible students, with the encouragement of modern Popes, have become much more conscious of the *gradualness* with which God gave His teaching in the Old Testament. They point out that an increasingly civilized moral consciousness came *only gradually* during centuries of God's teaching efforts, and that attitudes left over from pagan days were often tolerated or accepted unthinkingly by Abraham and other great leaders of the Israelites.

These attitudes are often simply recorded in the Jewish Scriptures without necessarily being endorsed by the Lord. Jesus alluded to this in mentioning Moses' toleration of divorce (Mt. 19:7). Contemporary Bible students point out also that the actual text of certain ancient formulations is not always immediately or easily clear to us in its precise meaning. For instance, in what sense do we understand "call" and "said" when we read, "God *called* to Abraham . . . and *said:* Take your son Isaac . . . and offer him up as a holocaust"? (Gn. 22:1–14).

Over the centuries the Church has developed a more and more accurate understanding (this is what "theology" helps the Church do) of what certain mysterious passages in the Bible mean. All of these unavoidable perplexities have simply been a stimulus for the Church to ponder more deeply and with greater conviction her vision of innocent human life as ultimately morally inviolable.

In the Bible inviolability of the innocent stands side by side with capital punishment and killing in warfare. The Exodus command, "The innocent and the just you shall not put to death," (Ex. 23:7) still speaks very firmly to innocent unborn human beings threatened by abortion and to those already born whose lives may be ended by suicide or euthanasia. This *Handbook* will return to these subjects in later chapters.

Challenges to the Individual

The doctrine of the individual human dignity and inviolability of innocent human persons faces two significant challenges from two strains of contemporary thinking. Both would minimize the uniqueness of each individual person.

One such idea is called pantheism (from the Greek—*pan*—"all"— and *theos*—"God": "All of us are nothing but a part of *God*.") Pantheism, which shows up both in certain Oriental religions and certain European philosophies, tends to consider the individual an "illusion" or "dream."

Another such system of thought, related to pantheism, is the materialistic version of evolution. This version omits the spiritual dimension of human beings entirely. It considers human persons to be purely material or organic creatures. All theories of evolution, it should be noted, need not be materialistic. Another kind of evolutionary theory, espoused by some scholars, admits of a historical process of evolution which produced ever more advanced creatures who, at some point in history, become human in and through a transformation and spiritualization.

Materialistic evolution tries to compare the whole human race to a kind of tree. In a tree the life which the trunk has is the same life which the branch has. Materialistic evolution (and other forms of materialism as well) would say that the life which the human race has is the same as the life which the individual person has. Hence, the individual person has no life or value except as part of the race—for the sake of what he contributes to the race.

Unfortunately, the tree theory destroys individual autonomy and inviolability. This means that the dignity and value of the tree's life as a whole outweighs any loss of life to a branch which may be pruned away for the tree's benefit. Individuals in such a theory are at least theoretically subordinated to the state or the nation. This represents essentially the theory which Pius XII rejected, as we noted above.

Living Longer—At What Price?

The Church's basic conviction, then, is quite clear:

(1) No one *can* ever destroy the *right* to life of an innocent person. Some may *try* to destroy that right, some may *claim* to destroy it. But in an innocent person, the right to life remains, even when it is violated.

(2) No one can ever be morally justified in *aiming* to take the life of an innocent person (including one's self). For an innocent person remains in the image of God.

But does this conviction mean also that I must therefore aim at the good *directly opposite* to killing? Does it mean that I must *prolong* human life, no matter what the circumstances? Must I always aim to *keep* myself or another *alive?*

Over the centuries, the Church has had a long, hard look at such questions. She has seen from the beginning, but with ever increasing clarity, that the answer is no! While the right to life does mean that *generally* I must take any steps necessary to preserve my own life or that of another, it does not *always* mean this. The Church recognizes what common intelligence also tells us: Sometimes we try to keep someone alive for the wrong reasons. Among these wrong reasons are: an abnormal unwillingness to face death as, in the end, unavoidable; a misguided scientific curiosity as to how long a dying person can be kept "alive"; or, in some cases, the professional pride of a physician who does not want to admit defeat. The great English poet Alexander Pope spotted these human foibles 300 years ago when he wrote:

> Thou shall not kill, yet needs't not strive
> Officiously to keep alive.

"Officiously," of course, means to take too seriously one's own "office" in life—the power God has given him—and to extend it beyond anything which God has granted to mere human beings.

Thus, if the price for prolonging life is agonizing physical pain, or financial ruin for one's family, or separation from one's home and loved ones (all with the hope of perhaps a few more hours, days, or weeks of breathing), then a sick man has a right to answer for himself the question: Is the price too high? And if he decides that it is, then he may rightly and without further medical resistance, let death come naturally when it will, as long as no one does anything aimed at actually producing death by either commission or omission.

The Church has also seen that the price of prolonging life may be too high if it keeps us from doing something good of immense value and necessity. Thus if certain drugs will kill the pain of a patient already terminally ill with cancer, but will also effectively cause some shortening of his life, then we may do what we have a right to aim to do (kill the pain), even though something else will result which we have *no* right to aim to do (shorten life). Or we may, similarly, remove a dangerously cancerous womb, even though the fetal life within it will perish as a result. The Church sees that there can be an enormous moral difference between *aiming* to cause death and *tolerating* its coming.

Recognizing at certain times, then, the futility of prolonging life, and at other times the impossibility of doing so, can be entirely compatible with recognizing the inviolability of innocent human life. But the essential principle still stands: one may never aim to destroy the life of an innocent person by either commission or omission.

Discussion Questions

1. Are there people today who show that they do not see anything sacred about the human body?
2. In what ways do people show their attitudes about their bodily life?
3. What teachings of the Church must we consider when we form our own opinions on capital punishment?
4. Is there bound to be any improvement in the Church's understanding of what it means for the life of the individual to be sacred?
5. Some political systems of the present day have been strongly influenced by materialistic evolutionism. What could one expect to happen in such systems to an individual who was judged to be an obstacle to the progress of that society?
6. In the teaching of the Catholic Church, does the sacredness of human life mean that every effort medically possible must be made to prolong life?

Preview of Chapter 5

- Dr. Raymond Adamek has analyzed public opinion research on abortion, euthanasia, and suicide.

- He found that survey wording can make a great difference in results, but opinion on the moral wrong of abortion is sharply divided.

- However, a majority of the respondents only approve of 5–10% of the abortions currently taking place in the United States, and the support for a Human Life Amendment ranges from 22% to 45%.

- News journalists, prominent educators, top federal officials, and leading lawyers are far more permissive about abortion than the general public.

- General approval of euthanasia increased by 61% over the past 30 years. One's attitude toward abortion and suicide will strongly predict one's attitudes toward euthanasia.

- But the American public is more willing to approve euthanasia than suicide, and less frequent attendance at religious services predicts greater permissiveness about euthanasia, suicide, and abortion.

CHAPTER 5

Public Opinion on Life Issues

The U.S. Supreme Court decisions of 1973 legalized most abortions of unborn human beings—removing that class of individuals from the "inviolability" discussed in the previous chapter. Many people feel that this will eventually lead to legalized mercy killing, at first of persons who request it, and eventually of other persons whose lives are judged by others as meaningless or excessively burdensome.

Is public opinion leaning in this direction? Do people really believe that the Supreme Court decisions on abortion were correct? Do the influential journalists and television commentators really have a pro-abortion bias?

An old proverb says, "Even the devil can quote Scripture to his own advantage." The numerous popular opinion polls about abortion and euthanasia are often quoted to the advantage of those approving these practices.

A professional sociologist from Kent State University in Ohio, Dr. Raymond J. Adamek, has analyzed most of the opinion polls about life issues of the past decade.[1] He has discovered that the largest percentage of the American people believe human life begins at conception. The majority have serious disagreements with the Supreme Court decisions on abortion and are generally closer to a pro-life than the so-called pro-choice perspective. This chapter will summarize Dr. Adamek's research.

The Acceptability of Abortion

The difficulty of accurately gauging public opinion on abortion can be clearly seen from three examples of poll questions where the response differed greatly depending on the wording. In Table 1, only 29% of the responses support an amendment to the Constitution to prohibit abortion, but 50% support an amendment to protect the life of the unborn child. Likewise, 64% agreed that the decision to have an abortion should be made solely by the woman and her physician, while only 24% thought a woman should be able to get an abortion without her husband's consent! While 44% opposed a woman going to a doctor to "end a pregnancy," 54% opposed going to a doctor "for an abortion."

Dr. Adamek compared eight different polls on the morality of abortion. He found proportions from 44% to 65% agreeing that abortion is morally wrong, with 41% finding it murder and 45% agreeing it is the equivalent of murder.[2] The ambivalence of many persons was evident in that up to 11% responded "don't know," "not sure," or "no opinion." But the clearly divided public opinion helps explain the considerable furor that has arisen over abortion legislation and court decisions.

At least seven different studies agree that approval for abortion in various circumstances increased between the early 1960's and the early 1970's in the U.S., and then levelled off after a final spurt following the Supreme Court's 1973 decisions.[3] A series of Gallup polls from 1975 to 1981 indicates that about 21 percent of adult Americans believe abortion should be illegal in all circumstances, and 23% believe it should be legal in any circumstance. Gallup discovered that a middle majority of respondents (52–55 percent) believe that abortion should be legal only for "hard reasons" (if the woman's life is endangered, or in cases of severe threats of health damage to the woman, or rape/incest) and only in the first three months (first trimester) of pregnancy.[4]

---

[1]See especially Dr. Adamek's publication "Abortion and Public Opinion in the United States" published April 22, 1982 by *NRL News*, Suite 402, 419 7th St. N.W., Washington D.C. 20004; reprints available.

[2]See above, Table 2.

[3]See above, notes 5–11.

[4]See above, Table 4.

Table 1. The Effect of Question Wording on Response: Three Examples

Responses*

A. Questions Regarding a Human Life Amendment

1. "Do you think there should be an amendment to the Constitution prohibiting abortions, or shouldn't there be such an amendment?"

	Should Be	Shouldn't Be
	29	67

2. "Do you believe there should be an amendment to the Constitution protecting the life of the unborn child, or shouldn't there be such an amendment?"

	50	39

B. Questions Regarding the Abortion Decision

1. "As you may have heard, in the last few years a number of states have liberalized their abortion laws. To what extent do you agree or disagree with the following statement regarding abortion: The decision to have an abortion should be made solely by a woman and her physician?"

	Agree	Disagree
	64	31

2. "Do you think it should be lawful for a woman to be able to get an abortion without her husband's consent?"

	Yes	No
	24	67

C. Questions Regarding the Supreme Court Decisions of 1973

1. "The U.S. Supreme Court has ruled that a woman may go to a doctor to end a pregnancy at anytime during the first three months of pregnancy. Do you favor or oppose this ruling?"

	Favor	Oppose
	47	44

2. "The U.S. Supreme Court has ruled that a woman may go to a doctor for an abortion at any time during the first three months of pregnancy. Do you favor or oppose this ruling?"

	43	54

*All responses in this and subsequent tables will be given in percentages. Figures may not add to 100 percent because of rounding, or because the "Other," "Don't Know" and "No Answer" responses have been omitted. See footnote 15 for Sources of these polls.

The middle majority would, in this Gallup study, approve abortion beyond the first trimester only when a mother's life is threatened. This leads Dr. Adamek to the important conclusion *that the middle majority of American people only approve 10 percent (and perhaps only 5 percent) of the legal abortions currently taking place in the United States.* This suggests grass roots disagreement with the public policy molded by the landmark abortion decisions of the Supreme Court in 1973.

Attitudes Toward the Supreme Court Decisions

The decisions of 1973 approved abortion on request through the first two trimesters of pregnancy. They allowed the states to forbid abortion in the third trimester except where it is necessary, in appropriate medical judgment, for the preservation of the life *or health* of the mother. The Court then gave a broad definition of health which, in effect, legalized abortion in the third trimester as well.

Both Harris and Gallup polls surveyed opinion about the Court decisions and found more approval than disapproval. But Adamek has ably argued that both polls focussed only on the court's legalization of abortion *in the first trimester*—an inaccurate way to test response to the real decisions.[5]

In fact, as already cited, other Gallup polls show 21% of the respondents opposing all abortions and the middle majority who would admit some abortions, limiting them to the first trimester except to save the life of the mother. *Hence the majority of the U.S. public does not approve the very permissive outcome of the 1973 Supreme Court decisions.*

Underlying this dissatisfaction with the Court decisions, one finds the basic question, "When does human life begin?" The Supreme Court's stated position was that it did not know when human life began. It appears, however, that the Court favored "viability" as the beginning of human life. It legalized all abortions in the first two trimesters when the fetus can be considered still not viable, or able to survive on its own. Since the Court also permitted abortions for "health" reasons in the third trimester, it even cast doubt on the full human dignity of the fetus until actual birth.

Dr. Adamek, on the other hand, has assembled four opinion polls where the belief that human life begins at conception is favored by 36% to 58% of the respondents.[6] The three polls in 1981 indicate that a ma-

---

[5]See above, Table 6 and Adamek, Raymond J., "Comment on Abortion Polls," *Public Opinion Quarterly*, 42:411–413.

[6]See above, Table 7.

jority of the public believes that human life begins within the first trimester, while only 5–17% believe it begins only when the baby is born.

Predictably, Gallup has demonstrated a strong relationship between one's beliefs about when life begins and the appropriate legal status of abortion. Thus, only 11% of those who believe human life begins at conception believe abortion should be legal in all cases, but 44% of those who believe it begins at birth feel that way.[7]

Dr. Adamek also cites data showing that only 20–35% of Americans agreed with the Supreme Court's 1976 decision that a married woman should be able to get an abortion without her husband's consent. The closest the Court and the American public come to agreement on abortion policy seems to be on the issue of using tax funds to pay for abortions. The Court in 1977 decided that neither federal nor state governments had to provide tax money for elective abortions. *Public opinion polls generally indicate majority support for this decision.*[8]

Hence, Adamek is wary of numerous polls he cites which seem to approve strongly the Supreme Court position of allowing abortion to be a private decision between a woman and her physician. He has shown that these polls generally tend to reflect a pro-abortion bias.[9] *In fact, the support for a Human Life Amendment indicates that a notable minority of the American public completely repudiates the Supreme Court decisions of 1973.*

Attitudes Toward Prohibiting Abortions

Since the "middle majority" of all Americans described above believe that abortion should be legal, but generally only in the first trimester, one can expect opposition to prohibiting all abortions. In fact, a review of national polls from 1978 through 1981 indicates that from 49% to 71% of Americans say they oppose, and from 22% to 45% say they favor, a Constitutional amendment to prohibit abortion.[10] However, *the support for an amendment is significantly greater than the 21% of the respondents in the Gallup polls who believe abortion should be illegal in all circumstances!*

Dr. Adamek believes that recent research has begun to uncover an explanation why this is so. He cites a study by Blake and Del Pinal

---

[7]Gallup, George, 1981, "Public Evenly Divided on 1973 Decision," *The Gallup Report* (July) Report No. 190:18–22.

[8]See above, Table 8.

[9]See above, Dr. Adamek's analysis of Table 9.

[10]Market Opinion Research, 1981, "Voters' Attitudes About Government Involvement in the Abortion Issue." (Nov. 18) 1–19.

which shows that a large group of respondents to some 18 abortion polls can be called "equivocators" and even "closet negatives" (i.e., closet anti-abortionists) in their views on legalizing abortion.[11]

Another current study shows that the general public is closer to pro-life activists than to pro-abortion leaders on 30 of 37 individual attitude items involving ethical judgment.[12] *Hence there is reason to believe that leaders of the pro-life movement more accurately reflect the ethical values of the American public than pro-choice activists.* This may indicate why the pro-life movement seems to be winning increasing support in its bid to protect human life by adding a positive affirmation to the Constitution itself.

Dr. Adamek has analyzed polls which contrast attitudes on abortion of people of different educational backgrounds, religious persuasion, geographic location, income, age, and sex. He has ranked the way in which different groups of people view abortion according to these groupings. In his list the first and strongest predictor of abortion attitudes is that those who attend religious services less frequently are more permissive about abortion than those who attend more frequently. Likewise, those with more formal education are more permissive than those with less formal education. Those who live in the East or West and those with higher incomes are more permissive than those living in the Midwest and South and those having lower incomes.

An interview study of 240 news journalists and broadcasters cited by Adamek indicated that these individuals represented a heavy concentration of persons who are predictably permissive on abortion because of their background. For example, they are not frequent in attending religious services and have comparatively high incomes and education. In fact, 79% of the three-fourths who responded did agree strongly with the statement that "a woman has a right to decide for herself whether to have an abortion." Another study reflecting the permissive attitudes on abortion by "opinion-makers" is the 1981 Connecticut Mutual Life Insurance poll which *found that 65% of the general public consider abortion morally wrong, but only 35% of the news media leaders feel that way. Furthermore, only 26% of prominent educators, 29% of top federal officials, and 25% of leading lawyers feel abortion is morally wrong!*

Of the four major religious categories usually analyzed in survey research (Protestant, Catholic, Jewish, and None), Catholics consistently have been found to be the least permissive toward abortion. Like others,

---

[11]Blake, Judith and Del Pinal, Jorge H., 1981, "Negativism, Equivocation, and Wobbly Assent: Public 'Support' for the Pro-choice Platform on Abortion," *Demography.* 18:309–320.

[12]Granberg, Donald and Denny, Donald, 1982, "The Coathanger and the Rose: Comparison of Pro-Choice and Pro-Life Activists in the Contemporary U.S.," *Transaction/Society* 19: 4:39–46.

Catholics have been becoming more permissive within the past two decades, apparently affected in generally the same way by the same social forces which affect others. Some evidence indicates that Catholics, especially younger Catholics, have become more permissive at a somewhat faster rate than the general public. A 1980 study by Granberg and Granberg found that, like other Americans, Catholics who were more permissive toward premarital sex, extramarital sex, homosexuality, and euthanasia were also more permissive toward abortion.[13]

Consistently, those Catholics who identified themselves as "strong Catholics" were less permissive toward abortion than not very strong Catholics. For example, Dr. Adamek has studied some 1980 data showing that only 18% of strong Catholics endorsed six or seven abortion justification items, whereas 42% did so of those who said they were not very strong Catholics. In this poll, 46% of those who identified themselves as Catholic stated that they attended religious services once a month or less. Frequency of attendance at religious services will also correspond closely to less permissive attitudes on euthanasia.

Attitudes Toward Euthanasia

Because abortion involves taking human lives which are unwanted or likely to suffer hardship, it has been called prenatal euthanasia. Will increasing acceptance of abortion lead to increasing acceptance of euthanasia? Table 2 has been prepared from several surveys which asked the same question. Although the question might conceivably be read to approve only withdrawing extraordinary means of prolonging life, its more literal reading asked *about mercy killing in an active sense.*

Two interesting facts in Table 2 are that while general approval of euthanasia increased by about 61% over the roughly 30 year period of the survey, *approval by Catholics increased by 100% and approval by those under 30 increased by 77%.* On the other hand, approval by Jews increased only 33%.

Dr. Adamek cites detailed analyses of these polls which show, as in the case of abortion, that those who attend religious services less frequently are more permissive about euthanasia than those who attend more frequently. In fact, while 40% of those who considered themselves

---

[13]Granberg, Donald and Granberg, Beth Wellman, 1980, "Abortion Attitudes, 1965–1980: Trends and Determinants," *Family Planning Perspectives* 12:250–261.

Table 2. Trends in Public Opinion on Euthanasia

Question: "When a person has a disease that cannot be cured, do you think doctors should be allowed by law to end the patient's life by some painless means if the patient and his family request it?" (Percent responding, "Yes".)

		1947	1950	1973	1977	1978
Total Sample:		36	36	53	59	58
Sex:	Men	—	38	53	65	62
	Women	—	34	53	55	55
Age:	Under 30	—	39	67	70	69
	30–49	—	37	51	58	58
	50 and over	—	30	44	53	49
Education:	Grade School	—	31	39	52	50
	High School	—	39	54	62	60
	College	—	42	61	67	66
Religion:	Catholic	28	—	48	60	56
	Protestant	36	—	53	57	55
	Jewish	54	—	60	71	72
	None	—	—	—	80	79

Sources: 1950 and 1973 data: *The Gallup Opinion Index* (August, 1973), Report 98, pp. 35–37; 1947 data: Ostheimer, John M. 1980, "The Polls: Changing Attitudes Toward Euthanasia," *Public Opinion Quarterly* 44:123–128. Source of 1977 and 1978 data: Davis, James A. 1980, *General Social Surveys 1972–1980*, Chicago: National Opinion Research Center. A dash indicates data are not available.

"strong Catholics" agreed with the euthanasia questions, 78% who considered themselves "not very strong" Catholics agreed. Protestants and Catholics, although different from one another in the earlier polls, are in the latter ones increasingly alike.

Two other variable factors are even stronger predictors of one's attitude toward euthanasia than the frequency of attendance at religious services. *These two factors are the person's attitude toward abortion and suicide, in that order.* This correlation tends to support the contention mentioned at the beginning of this chapter that permissive attitudes to abortion can lead the way to permissive attitudes toward euthanasia and suicide. This trend may become more noticeable as media attention and legal controversy focus increasingly upon euthanasia and suicide.

Russell Ward analyzed the 1977 National Opinion Research Center poll on euthanasia and discovered another significant fact.[14] In conducting an analysis on the respondents over the age of 60, he found that a person's own satisfaction with life can predict attitudes toward euthanasia. Persons with poor subjective health and low income are less satisfied with life than those who are more fortunate and also appear to approve euthanasia more readily.

Suicide

Dr. Adamek has found less public opinion data on suicide than on euthanasia, which in turn is much less than the data on abortion. He has analyzed a Gallup poll conducted in 1975 which focuses on suicide in cases of persons suffering great pain, or an incurable disease, or persons causing heavy burdens for their family. This might be called "mercy self-killing." *He finds the American public less willing to approve suicidal mercy killing than euthanasia administered by a doctor.* The approval comparison shows a 41% approval of suicidal mercy killing and a 59% approval of doctor-administered mercy killing.

Variables that predict respondents' attitudes toward abortion and euthanasia are good predictors of attitudes toward suicide as well. For example, frequent attendance at religious services predicts a low degree of permissiveness toward suicide. Thus 84% of the Catholics who say they attend religious services once a week show low approval of suicide, compared to 57% of those who say they attend once a month or less. *Likewise, of course, permissive attitudes on abortion and euthanasia will predict permissive attitudes on suicide.*

Conclusion

The data reviewed in this chapter leave room for some differences of interpretation. In some cases the data should be more complete. (For example, the data on Catholics are based on the responses of the 325–425 persons who are Catholic within the total national sample, instead

---

[14]Ward, Russell A., 1980, "Age and Acceptance of Euthanasia," *Journal of Gerontology* 35:421–431.

of a national sample of Catholics.) However, four conclusions about American attitudes toward critical life issues today stand out clearly:

1) *Attitudes toward abortion, euthanasia, and suicide are strongly interrelated.* Persons who are willing to accept deliberate killing as a means of solving personal and social problems in one of these contexts tend to accept it in all three contexts. *Thus, one may identify a pro-death ideology as well as a pro-life ideology in the United States today.*

2) *Church attendance and self-perceived strength of religious conviction are major determinants of where people stand in relation to the pro-life or pro-death ideology.* Catholics, particularly young Catholics, may have shifted toward the pro-death ideology somewhat more rapidly than persons of other religious groups. The fact that, in 1980, 38% of Catholics who attended religious services once a week or more could approve of euthanasia, sharply demonstrates that *Catholic teaching on euthanasia has either not been clearly learned or fully accepted.*

3) *The pro-death ideology has been gaining ground in the United States in recent years.* Dr. Adamek documented that trend in comparative studies on abortion and euthanasia attitudes. Other statistical evidence could be found in the yearly increase in the number of abortions, and perhaps in the frequency of deaths like that of Baby Doe in Bloomington, Indiana (See Chapter 14 and 15.)

4) *The data indicate some reluctance by those who have moral opposition to the pro-death ideology to support legal efforts to control the killing of human beings.* Apparently the fear of "imposing one's morality on others" has created this reluctance. Yet persons who believe in a pro-life ideology must actively support their convictions within the public life and political process of a free, democratic society. *Otherwise their silence actually supports the adoption of the pro-death ideology.*

Discussion Questions

1. In what ways does public opinion not approve of the Supreme Court decisions on abortion?
2. What is a pro-death ideology?
3. Why has the pro-death ideology gained ground in the United States in recent years?
4. Do poll results indicate what people themselves would actually do in circumstances where abortion, suicide, or euthanasia were contemplated?
5. Do the poll results indicate that religious ethics have a significant influence in the U.S. today?

6. Why are those who live in the East and West of the United States more permissive on abortion than those who live in the Midwest and the South?

---

[15]*Source of Question A:* New York Times/CBS News Poll. *The New York Times.* August 18, 1980, p. 1. Both questions were asked of the same respondents. *Source of Question B:* Question 1 was commissioned by Planned Parenthood and asked in a Gallup poll. *The Gallup Opinion Index,* Report 87, Sept. 1972. Question 2 was commissioned by Blake and asked in a Gallup poll two months after Question 1. Blake (1973) "Elective Abortion and Our Reluctant Citizenry," in Howard Osofsky and Joy D. Osofsky, *The Abortion Experience.* Maryland: Harper and Row. *Source of Question C:* Question 1: Gallup poll conducted March, 1974. *The Gallup Opinion Index,* Report 106, April 1974. Question 2: Sindlinger, "Special Hitchhiker on Abortion," for *National Review,* May 1974.

Preview of Chapter 6

- Suffering means much more than physical pain or discomfort.

- Dr. Cassel describes suffering as "the state of severe distress associated with events that threaten the intactness of the person."

- Critical illness affects different persons differently according to their background and outlook, and the kind of understanding health care they receive.

- But for everyone critical illness emphasizes the contingency and fragility of life and health. It challenges the spirit and affects all our relationships with "significant others."

- The Bible does not teach *why* people suffer, but it does teach *how* to suffer—in faith and hope and love.

- Pastoral care of suffering people can assist them to transcend their own weakness through the "redeeming grace" of Christ.

CHAPTER 6

A Pastoral Theology of Suffering

The first three chapters of this volume pictured the human person from several different perspectives and the next chapter discussed the inviolability of the life of an innocent human person. In contrast, the fifth chapter presented public opinion on the practices of abortion, euthanasia, and suicide, which directly and intentionally destroy innocent human lives.

Why take innocent lives? What element of common human experience could possibly explain this? Sometimes the answer is: human suffering. Sometimes human persons reach a point at which they believe they or someone loved by them would be better off dead than continuing to suffer. *This chapter will reflect upon suffering.*

Suffering means many things. We often describe ourselves as "suffering" when we are in pain or enduring some physical discomfort. It is not uncommon to speak of suffering of whole groups of people in a variety of different situations. We use the concept of suffering to describe the situation of the poor, the aged, the starving, and the sick. As contemporary Americans, we look at all of this suffering—usually from a distance—and remain grateful that we ourselves are not part of it. We try to keep our distance and leave the involvement in suffering to the physician, the medical technologist, and the politician.

Because of suffering, medicine and technology are assigned special positions in our culture. The doctor is seen as the gladiator or champion in the struggle against the suffering inflicted on mankind. The instruments of modern medical technology are his swords in the fight to rid mankind of the suffering caused by pain and disease. The spectacular success of medical technology has helped create this heroic image of the doctor. *People have come to believe that what modern medicine and technology cannot now cure will eventually be cured through more study, research, and technical advances.*

North Americans, with the exception of African Americans, hispanics, and native Americans, have not generally suffered in the way most of the world's poor suffer. They have lived in a land of plenty and have both the means and the opportunities to take advantage of the possibilities the resources provide. The suffering of the poor is seen as a public welfare problem whose solution belongs to politicians. Little thought and concern is given to the particular significance of this kind of suffering which crushes human self-respect. Consequently, politicians are simply mandated to rid society of poverty, rather than to develop strategies for healing its wounds.

Unfortunately, the effort to remove suffering from our existence has led to inadequate and inappropriate ways of dealing with it. For instance, our doctors are no longer those who care for the sick in their homes, but rather the high priests of healing enshrined in the temple of technology. And our politicians have become the cosmetologists of the human environment—trying to use a "band-aid" approach to remedy social injustices.

The Person Who Suffers

Why do human persons suffer? *The New England Journal of Medicine* published a special article on March 18, 1982, entitled: "The Nature of Suffering and the Goals of Medicine."[1] In this article, Eric J. Cassel, MD, defines suffering as *"the state of severe distress associated with events that threaten the intactness of the person."*

Doctor Cassel indicates that the cause of suffering is a state of severe distress. This is an extremely important point. Suffering need not be sickness or pain; it can be stress, guilt, a handicap, or many other

---

[1]Vol. 306, pp. 639–645.

feelings or situations. It is a state of being in which the integrity of the person is threatened.

Doctor Cassel has treated hundreds of suffering persons. *From his own medical expertise, he has concluded that suffering is an experience of persons and is not simply the physical pain they endure.* Suffering extends beyond the physical or biological order. Acute pain, shortness of breath, or other bodily symptoms tell the physician that a person is suffering, but the symptom is not the reality.

When the philosopher, René Descartes (1596–1650), analyzed human nature, he considered mind and body as two distinct realms. Thought characterizes the mind, whereas the body is noted for its "extension," its physical and material qualities. Doctor Cassel points out that, as medical science developed, it concentrated on the human body. The notion of "person" was synonymous with "mind" and was off limits to science.[2]

This meant that both mind and person were aspects of the human being that medicine did not consider in its earlier history. "Suffering," in this situation, was either *bodily pain* or it was *subjective*, in the mind, and not truly "real."

Today, though, one can literally say that "suffering is ultimately a personal matter."[3] Persons are neither simply bodies or simply minds. Persons are mind/body individuals, and suffering is a mind/body experience.

One instance of the mind's influence on bodily pain cited by Doctor Cassel concerned a woman with severe pain in her leg. As long as she believed it to be caused by sciatica, a pain arising from the sciatic nerve, she could control her pain with small doses of codeine. When she discovered that the pain was due to a spreading malignancy, much greater amounts of pain medication were necessary.

Other "personal" aspects of suffering affect the degree of pain one reports. For instance, a person with kidney stones will endure extreme pain rather calmly as long as he or she "knows what it is." Fear that their pain will become uncontrollable can lead terminal cancer patients to report unendurable pain. If that fear is removed by the administration of effective pain-killing medication, these patients will often be able to tolerate subsequent pain with less medication or none at all. They find that they can handle the "controllable" pain and may even prefer it to the side effects of the medication.

Hence physical pain will affect persons differently according to how they perceive the pain in relation to their own continued existence and their own well-

---

[2]*Ibid,* p. 640.
[3]*Ibid.*

being as persons. That's why Doctor Cassel included in his description of suffering the "events that threaten the intactness of the person."

This volume has already presented several chapters on the person as understood in modern thought. A core theme thus far has been the interaction of body and soul or spirit which occurs within the individual life story of every living person. Reflections found in this chapter on suffering as a personal experience support this theme. Persons suffer even without pain, and persons can endure pain without really suffering. The mind and body continuously interact. Normally, of course, critical illness brings both pain and suffering.

Suffering and Critical Illness

Suffering, taken in Doctor Cassel's sense of the state of severe distress associated with events that threaten the intactness of the person, will normally accompany critical illness, whether or not physical pain is present. _But every person suffers in his or her own particular way._ Some individuals, for example, have prided themselves on their self-sufficiency. They suffer more acutely in critical illness than others who are accustomed to depending on others. One's cultural and ethnic background may dictate whether visitors are welcome during critical illness. A person who is secure in a strong and happy marriage can handle critical illness better than someone in a marriage that is falling apart. A person who has successfully survived in a previous critical illness will often be better able to tolerate critical illness than someone who was "never sick a day in his life."

Similarly, a person suffering the same critical illness which others in the family have experienced will often be better able to cope with it. Persons who are able to understand the diagnosis and prognosis of their illness because of kind and sensitive explanations by physicians and nurses will suffer less than others, even if the pain is the same. Persons who pride themselves on physical strength or attractiveness will suffer more from the same weakening or disfiguring illness than others who pay little attention to strength or appearance.

Despite these very personal factors in suffering, four common elements faced by everyone with a critical illness can be outlined.[4]

First, critical illness accentuates the contingency of human life, the unpredictable future everyone faces. For the sick person the possibility of death

[4]See "Sickness in a Christian Anthropology" by Francois H. Lepargneur O.P., _The Mystery of Suffering and Death_, edited by Michael J. Taylor S.J. (Staten Island, N.Y.,: Alba. House, 1973) pp. 71–81.

becomes a stark reality instead of a theoretical future event conveniently left in the recesses of the mind.

(a) *Secondly, critical illness increases awareness of the fragility of health and well-being.* Where before the person had given little thought to the blessing of health, now a deep sense of loss and even a kind of grief sets in.

(3) *Thirdly, the person experiencing critical illness finds new challenges to the human spirit and the power of freedom to triumph over the forces of nature and flesh.* The existentialist trend in modern thought emphasizes that each person chooses who they will be in the face of given circumstances. Will the sick person become depressed and self-centered? Or will the sick person summon inner strength and spiritual energy to maintain a calm and unruffled disposition? Sickness constricts bodily freedom and mobility, but the person can *freely* choose to transcend the obstacles by realistically assuming the burdens.

(4) *Finally, critical illness stirs up new aspects of a person's relationship to others, especially the "significant others" in his or her life.* While sickness tends to isolate the sufferer, it also makes one more dependent upon others. It affects all social relations, sometimes turning them sour through bitterness, jealousy, or pride. Sometimes it improves the depth and quality of relationships because of compassion and empathy.

These four themes suggest, collectively, that suffering can play an extremely constructive and positively beneficial role in the lives of individual persons. Yet a key to such growth and purification remains the freedom of the human spirit. How do people obtain the strength to transcend their own suffering and misfortune? Or should we speak of the redeeming grace which helps persons who suffer transcend their own weakness and helplessness? "Redeeming grace" suggests that faith and Biblical revelation should be consulted.

Faith and Biblical Revelation

Undoubtedly the best-known Old Testament discussion of human suffering is in the book of Job. Job presents us with the problem of suffering and man's inability to understand it. We see in Job the tragic suffering of a just man. Job, himself, tries to understand the "why" of his suffering, while his friends take their turns at accusing him of some wrongdoing that has caused his suffering.

The three friends of Job are trying to console him by defending the doctrine of retribution. According to the friends, Job must have strayed from the path of virtuous living at some time, and God is now giving Job his just desserts.

Job, however, could not accept the explanation of his friends. The doctrine of retribution found in the Wisdom books of the Bible could not satisfy Job in his mind or heart. He became angry with his friends and silenced them. As he lost his taste for life, he thought relief was possible only in death. Yet, even death was not a solution for Job. He demanded understanding and sought union with God.

The author of the Book of Job does not seem to be able to go any farther. God does come to Job, but does not answer the question "why?". *Perhaps the best the author could offer the believer was a faith that simply states that God has other purposes for suffering than merely the exercise of retributive justice.*

An obvious "other purpose" of suffering seen in the Old Testament is the purpose of challenging the suffering person, like Job or Jeremiah the prophet, to decide whether he or she would *accept or reject* a God who could mysteriously allow suffering without apparent reason. Jeremiah struggled with this very decision, but always, in the end, placed his trust in God. Certainly it was in part his suffering which caused him to become one of the greatest of the Old Testament prophets.[5]

Father Francis Clearly, S.J., a Biblical scholar, has outlined some eight ways in which the Old Testament interprets suffering. He includes a sacrificial role when suffering serves as a means of reconciliation with God (Is. 40–55). Another role he notes is eschatological—the way suffering contributes to the coming of the end time when God will bring forth final deliverance (Is. 4–27).[6]

In later Judaism there developed a world view which held that God would conquer death. Christ, the long-awaited hero of the New Testament, "has robbed death of its power and brought life and immortality into clear light through the gospel." (2 Tim. 1:10) In the promise of the Bible, "He shall wipe every tear from their eyes, and there shall be no more death or mourning, crying out or pain, for the former world has passed away." (Rev. 21:4)

Christ accomplished His victory over death by assuming mortal nature and "sinful flesh." (Rm. 8:3) Death came into the world as punishment for sin. But for Christ it became a sign or love and submission to His Father. "I am the resurrection and the life," Jesus proclaims, "Whoever believes in me, though he should die, will come to life." (Jn. 11:25–26)

---

[5]See McCarthy, Rev. Donald G., *Care for Suffering and Dying Persons* (Washington, D.C., Bishops' Committee for Pro-Life Activities, 1978) pp. 8–10.

[6]Cleary S.J., Francis X., "Biblical Perspectives on Suffering," *Hospital Progress*. Dec. 1974, pp. 54–58. See also, *Genetic Counseling, The Church and the Law*. edited by Gary M. Atkinson and Albert S. Moraczewski O.P. (St. Louis: Pope John Center, 1980; Distributor for the Trade: Franciscan Herald Press, Chicago), pp. 80–85.

During His earthly ministry Jesus explained the necessity of the cross of suffering for all His followers. Thus, precisely after Peter's confession of Jesus as the Messiah, Jesus gave His disciples the lesson of the cross. (Mk. 8:27–38) "If a man wishes to come after me, he must deny his very self, take up his cross, and follow in my steps. Whoever would preserve his life will lose it, but whoever loses his life for my sake and the gospel's will preserve it." (vv. 34ff) *Jesus taught that there is no entrance into messianic glory without suffering.*

Jesus did not teach that all suffering is punishment for sin, the doctrine of retributive justice. For example, in the case of the man born blind, Jesus was asked whether the sin of that man or his parents had caused him to be born blind. "Neither," answered Jesus, "it was no sin, either of this man or of his parents. Rather is was to let God's work show forth in him." (Jn. 9:1–3)

Jesus frees us from the notion of God the avenger. Our God is not to be seen as the judge waiting to carry out his sentence. *Instead, he is the God who will trust his servant to serve him. God trusted Job to remain faithful and he did.* God trusted Jesus to be faithful and he was. In his fidelity to the Father, Jesus becomes the example for us of what it means to be faithful to the Father.

Suffering is part of the human condition, but need not be seen as a meaningless gesture or irrational act. Suffering becomes a meaningful act when accepted with the same mind as Christ. "All this is as God intends, for it is your special privilege to take Christ's part—not only to believe in him but also to suffer for him." (Phil. 1:28–29)

St. Paul spoke of his own suffering in this vein: "I wish to know Christ and the power flowing from his resurrection; likewise to know how to share in his sufferings by being formed into the pattern of his death. Thus do I hope that I may arrive at resurrection from the dead." (Phil. 3:10–11)

St. Paul also presents in the New Testament the possibility of vicarious suffering when he writes about the Church as the Body of Christ. This possibility was introduced in the well-known "Suffering Servant" poems of Isaiah, especially Isaiah 53. This involves a concept of corporate personality, whereby one person can, as it were, efficaciously represent others and suffer for their sins because of the union among the members of a covenant group.

Paul taught that because of the intimate union among the members of the Body of Christ and also between them and Christ, the actions of one can have an effect on the others. That is why he could write: "Even now I find my joy in the suffering I endure for you. In my own flesh I fill up what is lacking in the sufferings of Christ for the sake of his body, the church," (Col. 1:24)

Faith and Biblical revelation, then, do not explain *why* all instances of human suffering occur. But a clear doctrine emerges which teaches followers of Jesus *how* to give meaning to their suffering. The "redeeming grace" through which suffering Christians transcend their weakness and helplessness is the grace of Christ. It is in love of Him that Christians face suffering and death. St. Paul gave pastoral encouragement to suffering persons in his famous hymn of love. "There is no limit to love's forbearance," he wrote, "to its trust, its hope, its power to endure." (I Cor. 13:7)

Pastoral Care of Suffering Persons

Persons who suffer, as pointed out earlier in this chapter, experience more than physical pain; suffering affects persons in their whole being and threatens their intactness. Suffering persons need to "work through" the challenge of suffering in order to continue their journey through life.

The well-known author and psychiatrist, Doctor Viktor Frankl, teaches that "self-transcendence is the essence of existence." Every person must freely choose to search for the meaning of life in order to go beyond the meaningless. The Christian searches for meaning in the context and comfort of faith and Biblical revelation. *The Christian finds nobility, responsibility, and freedom in his or her relationship to Christ.*

Each human person is complete and unique. The individual is able to grow into some kind of fullness of being that is unlike that of any other person. Each person is a new creation of God and is called to witness the unfolding meaning of his existence. The pastoral minister must be acutely aware of these facts of completeness and uniqueness.

The person is a spiritual being. The person is more than an organism and has worth and dignity independent of useful qualities or functions. To see a person as less than spiritual runs the risk of seeing that person as an object. Psychoanalysis, for example, tends to regard the patient as ruled by mechanisms and the therapist as the one who knows how to handle these mechanisms.

Pastoral care shows a suffering person that he or she need not just be a helpless victim. A suffering person is capable of actualizing the values inherent in his life's situation. Confronted with the unalterable, something imposed by destiny, the patient becomes responsible for seeking a meaning in the situation. The person is ever in the process of becoming, of transcending the condition of suffering, of reaffirming his relationship to Christ and thus finding meaning in his or her being and

67

existence. This means that a human life can be fulfilled, not only in creating and enjoying, but also in suffering.

It is the pastoral minister's role to help the suffering person to find his or her meaning and value in the faith that is offered to us in the person of Jesus Christ. By accomplishing this, the person is free to transcend the otherwise meaningless suffering and find a oneness with the suffering Christ who is ever offering himself to the Father. This is a new meaning for the suffering person, who is now no longer the helpless victim, but the victim who triumphs over suffering and death.

The person who suffers for, with, and in Christ has understood the Word of God—both the Biblical Word and Jesus, the Incarnate Word. Such a person has taken responsibility for his or her human condition, and is prepared to enter ever more deeply into spiritual union with God and the human family. This person has entered consciously into the process of moving all creation to its fullness in a new heaven and a new earth.

The pastoral theology of suffering outlined here applies to persons experiencing inevitable suffering despite medical care and other forms of human care and comfort. This theology provides a faith-filled value system for confronting human suffering. Yet in the contemporary world where practices like abortion, euthanasia, or suicide offer quick and relatively painless solutions to human problems, this pastoral theology may seem fanciful or unrealistic.

But human persons are persons of dignity and destiny. The critical issues at the beginning of human life and in caring for human life discussed in the remainder of this volume must be seen in the light of that dignity and destiny.

Discussion Questions

1. How would you explain the difference between suffering and pain?
2. Why did medicine traditionally concentrate on bodily pain rather than suffering?
3. How can critical illness play a constructive and beneficial role in the lives of suffering persons?
4. What did St. Paul teach about vicarious suffering?
5. What does Dr. Frankl mean by saying that "self-transcendence is the essence of existence?"
6. Why does suffering with Christ offer a promise of triumph or victory?

PART TWO

Critical Issues at the Beginning of Human Life

Preview of Chapter 7

- One of the first things a human embryo does is to produce special cells, called gametes, which will enable it to be a parent many years later.

- Over the years, as the human embryo develops into a mature infant, then a new-born child, and finally a young adult, it harbors and cultivates the special gamete cells until they are ready to act as sperm or ova to beget a new human being.

- When a new human embryo begins, its body, even as a single cell, shows organization for eventually producing the brain and nervous system.

- These biological facts help us see the answer to the question: When does a truly new human being begin? When is this new being a *person*, with all the *basic rights* of a person?

- It is difficult, in a society of factions and controversy, to see the answer to these questions.

- The clue to the answer is whether and from what point in its existence a human embryo has something in it to organize it to do eventually all that a truly human body can do.

- God alone calls a person to be a person by giving that person the capacity to know and choose in a human way.

CHAPTER 7

The Beginning of a Life and a Person

The two boys, 11 and 12 years of age, didn't want to tell her but they did anyway. "Mom, 'Mikey' didn't do it. We did it."

"Mikey" was the two-year old who got blamed for breaking the lamp which now lay in pieces on the living room floor, and he would have gotten a mild, but significant slap on the fingers from his mother, had his two big brothers not owned up to the deed. The whole thing was an experience they would laugh about twenty years later. And, though "Mikey" was too little when it all happened to talk in terms of "person-hood" or "injustice" or "violation of rights," yet he was experiencing what those words stood for. For he had experienced: (1) that he was an individual distinct from his brothers, and could not be blamed (or praised) for what they did; and (2) that he had rights as much as any-body else, including the right not to be punished for something he hadn't done.

Perhaps at some time in your life *you* were a "Mikey"—or one of his older brothers. Ask yourself, then: When did you become an individual distinct from all other human beings? And *when* did you get the personal rights which belong to every human being? *When you were 11 or 12, or like "Mikey," only 2? Or when you were 1? Or the day you were born? or 3 or 6 or 8 months before that?*

A Biological Fact: Human Beings Call Other Entirely New Human Beings Into Existence

We all know that a sperm and ovum, each with its own set of chromosomes, combined to determine the kind of bodily life with which each of us would live in this world. We know that, because each of our parents provided only part of those chromosomes, we are not totally like either of them. Nor are we exactly like any other human being, because the path on which our inherited genes has sent us off is at least a little bit different from that of any other human being that ever has or ever will exist. All this is common knowledge.

A Beginning Life Aims Towards Another Beginning Life

What may not be so commonly known, however, is that the newly formed human embryo is, from its very first days, preparing itself to be a parent to another human embryo years later. It will produce another human being who, though equal in its basic human worth, will be an individual entirely distinct from its parent. We all know, it is true, that a new and healthily formed human being is marked as male or female from the day that an X or Y chromosome of the sperm combines with an X chromosome of the ovum. We know, too, that if this combination of sex-determining chromosomes is fostered by the right environment within the womb, the appropriate reproduction system of a female or a male child will begin to develop visibly—within eight weeks after conception, embryologists tell us. Thus the newly forming body is propelled towards one day being able to produce its own offspring.

What many of us do not know is that the cells which will become eventually sperm or ova do not wait even these eight weeks to appear. *Within four days* of conception, the hardly more than microscopic new embryo has succeeded in producing certain cells which will eventually become sperm or ova. These highly specialized cells (called gametes), different from all the cells with which the embryo is forming its *own* bones and tissues and organs, are structured to become the bones and tissues and organs of *another* embryo which will not be conceived until perhaps 15, or 20, or 30 years later. Present from at least four days after conception, these gamete cells, embryologists tell us, have migrated within four weeks, to the part of the developing embryo where the newly forming testes or ovaries are found. The arrival of the gametes at this point accelerates the development of the testes or ovaries. These organs in turn cause the gametes cells themselves to further complete their own internal self-structuring. *Thus, along with building up its own structure, one of the first things a new embryo does is to provide cells for the future existence of yet another entirely distinct human being.*

One Body Moves Towards Procreating Another

Years later, when this developing embryo is fully maturing, the gamete cells (or cells evolved from them) will undergo a final development into completed sperm or ova. One such development is a complicated process (meiosis) by which the gametes rid themselves of half their chromosomes, thus allowing for and even inviting combination with the chromosomes of a gamete from a member of the opposite sex. As the final development takes place, the ovum is extremely active within itself, producing (synthesizing) certain acids (RNA—Ribonucleic Acid) in the extraordinary quantities necessary to support a new embryo should the ovum be fertilized. Then — suddenly when the ovum reaches maturity — this and other rather exuberant activity inside the ovum comes to a complete halt. In other words, it comes to a halt precisely when the ovum has enough of what it needs to support the beginnings of life of another new human individual. Just as the ovum undergoes these dramatic changes, so also does the sperm cell, but only when it is released into the female generative organs and has managed to get quite close to the ovum. At this point, the front two thirds of the head of the sperm is softened (capacitation) as an outer layer is dissolved (acrosome reaction), making it possible for the sperm to penetrate the ovum.

With this penetration, the ovum, sleeping since it reached its optimum quota of RNA and the other chemicals it needs to support a new life, suddenly wakes up and begins to produce extraordinary quantities of proteins. The ovum also toughens its outer surface and makes other changes to prevent another sperm cell from entering into it.

These are just a few of the changes which take place in the mature ovum and sperm, especially as they meet. Just as the embryo produced gametes in its first days of existence so now the mature body which developed from that embryo propels itself toward producing a new human individual. It will be an individual with a combination of chromosomes never seen before and with resulting characteristics unique to itself alone.

The New Embryo: From the First, Cells Organized
Into a Unified Body

Once begun, this newly fertilized ovum, like all others, immediately begins to organize itself into an orderly body all its own. Its "right" and "left" are immediately established on each side of the place where the sperm entered the ovum, and from that point grows all the symmetry with which we are so familiar in our own bodies. Its "top" is established at the other end from the "bottom." These points of "length" and "width" being settled from the outset, the production of RNA and other chemicals increases at what will become the "back" of the newly fertilized ovum, while such syntheses is somewhat notably sparcer at the "front."

As the cells divide into new cells (mitosis), within a few days they trigger in one another a process by which they become cells different from one another, i.e., one group takes off on its own to develop nerve tissue; another, heart tissue; another bone cells, and so on. (From the fourth day, as we have noted above, some cells [gametes] move towards becoming sperm and ovum.) This process of cells' becoming different from one another is stimulated by chemicals in the mother's system, and cannot, once begun in a cell, be reversed.

Thinking Upon These Things

We have been reviewing in a summary way the means by which a new human being — as an embryo only a few days old, then as a developing fetus, and finally as a mature adult — provides the gamete cells. It is precisely these gamete cells which, *many years later as sperm and ovum*, are necessary for the beginning of yet another human being. These are biological facts accessible to the probings of the material senses of the scientist and to testing in the laboratory.

These biological facts about the way material cells act have meaning far beyond the purely physical; they stimulate our exploration of philosophical and theological facts as well. The biological facts lead us to think about the way existence overcame nothingness, about the reality of intelligent planning behind our universe. They cause us to ask whether human persons can detect the plans of an Intelligence, understand His decisions, and do their own planning and decision-making as well. We ask ourselves whether these biological facts take place this way because Someone deliberately plans it so.

The person who believes in God, of course, is convinced that the answer can be only: Yes! Such a person can recognize that his "Yes!" is not only the fruit of some childhood religious training; it is also an intellectually respectable and even compelling position. For the religious person, then, the acceptance of an ultimate Creator Who is ultimately over and above all else that exists is basic.

Basic too is the question of whether man can in any way enter into the mind of this Creator — understand His purposes. Convinced that he can deal and is dealing with a Creator Who is "speaking His mind" in all that he does, the believer in our scientific age looks at the biological facts of the inner and outer activity of the new embryo from its first days. The believer asks: Is this truly a *new and distinct human being* with an existence basically distinct from all others? And, if so, does this new being have all basic rights as a *person* from the first moment of its existence?

Philosophic Questions: We Can't Live With Them or Without Them

These are what we call, for want of a better term, "philosophic questions." Many persons have never, to their own satisfaction, answered the "philosophic question" of the existence of God. Yet these same people still try to face the "philosophic question" of the individual existence and personal rights of a human being.

We must remember, then, that it is always difficult to convince everyone on all issues simply by philosophic reasoning. This is true even when the arguments presented are really quite sound and convincing. It is true even among persons who are in basic agreement on many fundamental questions. It is true wheh fundamental questions of the meaning of life are being considered serenely and without bias.

It is especially and painfully true, however, in a society which is highly "Pluralistic" (this is often a polite term for "fragmented"), where many deny that there is or can be any meaning or sense to life, or any One to provide any hope for meaning or sense. Such a "pluralistic society" will find many in its ranks who deny or at least will not admit that there is such a thing as an individual human being truly distinct from the race as a whole, or truly raised, by dignity as a *person*, above the status of totally material animals.

The obstacles to uncovering any human meaning in the facts of embryo development and activity are multiplied, moreover, when a pluralism of views becomes impassioned and politicized, as in the case in the United States currently where the battle over abortion rages. "Politics" too easily degrades itself into getting what the most powerful want, and the *truth* about what is worthy of us or beneath us as human beings takes a back seat. "Passion", while good in itself, can become an emotionalism which short-circuits the thinking even of well-meaning persons.

Where the Believer Starts

In trying to uncover invisible truths which may shine through the visible biological facts of the human embryo's life, the believer begins already convinced as to certain basic realities. These convictions have not gone unexamined in the light either of keen rational thought or of theological testing. Christians trained in these mental disciplines find these beliefs in harmony with faith in Christ as the Catholic church has always known Him.

In the past five years, most of the older Protestant church bodies have seen the emergence of ever more vocal pro-life, anti-abortion groups within their own constituencies. A few of these traditional Protestant bodies are beginning to make official public statements offering at least some resistance to abortion. Newer, evangelically-oriented churches usually have strong pro-life commitments very close to those of the Catholic Church.

In some cases, these beliefs are also discoverable and defensible even by thinking persons who do not have Christian commitments. Indeed many of these truths are evident even to people who are uncertain as to the existence of God, but who are, nonetheless, allied in movements to defend human fetal life. (See Dr. Bernard Nathanson's testimony in his book, *Aborting America*). We would formulate these "starting points" as follows:

(a) The world *has meaning* and *makes sense*, and has One Who gives it this meaning and sense, inasmuch as He causes it to be. (This belief does not necessitate denying that meaninglessness and senselessness — in a word, evil — also are part of our world.)

(b) Sincere human thought is *able to uncover this meaning and sense* of created life, as well as the presence of Him Who creates them. (This belief does not deny that some may be hindered through no fault of their own from using their natural capacity to understand God's plan and presence.)

(c) Different things and especially persons have an existence as individuals. "I am not you, and you are not I." This individual existence is not a dream or illusion. (This does not deny that individuals are interdependent or must energetically adjust to the rest of reality.)

(d) Some material things are *forcefully organized* into being parts of a *living thing* (the chemicals and minerals that make up our bodies), while others merely *happen* to be drawn to each other (the stars and planets of our galaxies and our solar systems.)

(e) The *human being* is a *living material thing*, that is, an *organism*. This means that:

  (1) It tends to *maintain* its identity, organization, and composition against loss. (Homeostasis)

  (2) It depends on *relationships* for survival:
    —relationships between its own various parts
    —relationships with other entities distinct from itself.

  (3) It makes what *adjustments* it can and needs to in response to contact with other entities distinct from itself, as well as to changes within its own parts.

(f) The human person is an *embodied* being, i.e., there is no pre-existing soul which "comes into" a body and makes it human. The new existence of the soul and the new existence of the body are the same thing.

(g) As scientific knowledge about the structures of the human body continues to grow, we understand more and more deeply God's plan for us in our bodily life.

The Search for the Primary Organizer of the Truly Human Body

To begin functioning like a human being, a person must have a highly developed nervous system (what Aristotle and other early observers of human anatomy called the "power of inner sensation"). This highly developed nervous system makes possible the memory, the imagination and the flow of energy necessary for consciousness and decision-making. Without such a developed nervous system a body could never be called functionally "human," for it could not provide for activity typical of human beings.

The organ which produces this "power of the inner sensation" or nervous system is of primary importance if one is to have a truly "human" body. Which organ is it?

Aristotle, depending on the data recorded by physicians of his time, presumed that this "primary organizer" was the *heart*. The heart, the ancients thought, produced the "power of inner sensation," *the nervous system* and especially the central part of it, *the brain*. It was not a bad guess, given the state of anatomy and physiology in Aristotle's day. Indeed, there was not really another likely option available for his thinking. It was from this presumption that Aristotle, along with the "embryologists" of his day, drew the conclusion there was no truly *human* body until forty days after conception when, observations of miscarried fetuses had shown, a *heart* was present and able to function.

No scientist would doubt today, of course, that it is the *brain* which is the "primary organizer." When we have a functioning fetal brain, sending out its various signals to the rest of the body to propel forward the proper development of all its organs and systems, then we have the truly "primary organizer." It is at this point that we have a truly *human body*.

This fetal brain appears clearly at 8 weeks. But, if the brain is *a* primary organizer does that mean that it is the *only* primary organizer the human organism ever knows? If there is *another* primary organizer three or four or five weeks *before* the nervous system is present, then do we not at *that* point have a truly *human* body? Do we not at *that* point have a body containing a part which is capable of thrusting the whole organism forward towards complete development of the "power of inner sensation"?

Such indeed is the case. For, as one might expect, the brain does not just "appear," but is brought into existence by a "primary organizer" which *precedes* it, namely the *"primitive streak"* of nerve tissue which will develop into the brain. And before that, the "primitive streak" is brought into existence by the *organizing center* of the embryo's germinating (blastula) stage. And before that, by the *nucleus* of the fertilized ovum (unicellular zygote). Thus the argument is strong that from the instant in which that *nucleus* is formed by the fusion of the chromosomes of ovum and sperm, we have a *truly new human individual*. We have one whose body has a part (the nucleus) capable of propelling it towards the development of the high type of nervous system which is needed for truly human functioning. The nucleus, then, is the first of a series of "primary organizers" for the new human being.

"Good Men Differ . . ."

We have been focusing on the presence of a whole succession of "primary organizers," going back to the nucleus of the newly fertilized ovum. This nucleus *seems* to be the clear signal that a new and basically whole human being is present, for this nucleus is capable of programming the eventual development of the nervous system and especially the brain. This nervous system with its brain is the component essential to the body if it is to be a medium for the truly human and spiritual activity which we call intellect and will.

The nucleus, then, *seems* to mark the beginning of a truly human body. Some theologians and philosophers, however, question this conclusion. Although they have more accurate physiological data than did Aristotle and Aquinas, they would argue that no newly forming body is truly capable of being human for anywhere from two weeks to three months after conception. Accordingly, during this period (authors differ as to its length), there cannot possibly be, they would say, a new human person present in the womb.

"I Am a Body. Does That Count?"

The thinking Christian, then, would say that each one of us has a truly human body many months prior to birth, although, as we have seen, there is disagreement as to precisely at what point this is the case.

At least in our time, however, the thinking Christian is faced with another "philosophic question": Is it *enough* to have a truly human body? Is that enough to make me a *person*? The Catholic Church, in the conviction that she is being true to herself and to the truth about man as it is revealed in her knowledge of the person of Jesus Christ, answers unhesitatingly: Yes! In the face of such a "Yes!," the thinking Christian will examine three present-day answers to the "philosophic question": By *whose decision* can an individual be called a human person?

The three answers are these:

1) *God's decision*, conferring personhood from the first moment of conception.
2) *The person's own decision* by which he begins to act as a morally responsible agent.
3) *The decision of others*, as when society "confers" personhood on him.

Without denying that some elements of truth may indeed be present in each of these three answers, most people will see immediately that only the first one can be said to be in any *basic* sense compatible with the Church's position.

The first position is that personhood depends on the creative decision of God. The decision is literally "em-bodied" (put into a body) in the truly human embryo. And what makes an embryo truly human? Its internal capacity for whatever neurological activity is fundamental to the human way of knowing and choosing, which is to know and act *in and through the body and especially its neurological system.*

This neurological capacity may be ready at hand, as it normally is in each of us as an adult. It is "on call," available for our using at any moment we choose. Or this neurological capacity may even be "one step removed" from being "on call." For the human individual must be said truly to have this capacity if his body has the *capacity to produce the necessary neurological system*, even though the body may not yet have actually done so.

The main point of this approach is that I have a *capacity* for something whether or not I am *here-and-now* using that capacity. And it is the *capacity* for certain actions which makes me what I am — a human person. Thus, a sleeping man has the *capacity* for rational conversation, even though he may not be using it here-and-now. But he does not *lose* his basic status as a human person simply because, at this moment, he has an almost unused neurological capacity. For example, I cannot justify shooting him on the excuse that he is sleeping, and therefore not *using* his neurological capacity as a human being in any significant way.

There are, moreover, different *degrees* of neurological capacity. Some people are not as "intelligent" as others: that is they do not remember, recall, react as well. Does that make them less *persons*? No, this first approach must say. Nor does the *lowest of all degrees* of neurological capacity mean that we do not have a person. That *lowest* degree belongs to the newly fertilized ovum which has, locked in its nucleus, the internal power to produce its own truly human neurological system.

This first "philosophical" approach, then, would say that one's status as a person with all the rights of a person does not go "on" or "off" with the actual use or non-use of our capacity for consciousness. This status belongs to any human being with even a *capacity* — however undeveloped, damaged or dormant — for *any* degree of human consciousness.

The second approach to the question would say: I make myself a person by my own conscious thoughts and/or responsible decisions. This approach can be traced in various forms back at least to the 17th century philosopher Descartes and his "*Cogito ergo sum*": "I think, therefore I am." (Note how this contrasts with the Church's position, which says: No! Long *before* you think, you are! You are when your body gives you even the *capacity* to think or the potential to develop that capacity.)

This second position, in most recent times, says, in effect, that I must be able here-and-now to give and get *attention*. Proponents of this position sum up this requirement in the word "socialization." Anyone who is not capable of hearing others and making himself heard is, in effect, to be treated not as an acting person (a subject), but as a thing (an object). One writer with this approach will not admit that a human being is a person unless that human has a functioning brain, awareness of his own individuality, and a capacity for enjoying life and human relationships. He thus excludes the human fetus, as well as the comatose, the severely suffering, or the senile.

Another writer would allow for any *useful* killing of the fetus because it does not yet have full moral responsibility. He tries, however, to escape the logical application of his principle to "young children" by appealing to the third possible philosophic position, which we will now mention briefly.

This third position is that the decision of *others* makes us persons. Others, for serious reasons, "grant" or "attribute" personhood to us, with all its basic rights. Thus we as a society bestow personhood on young children (thus legally ruling out infanticide) because they are already undergoing *some* process of "socialization." In contrast, we have no serious reasons for "bestowing personhood" on the unborn.

Once Upon A Time Jesus Was A Human Embryo

It seems necessary to say the Church's position on this issue is not rooted only or even primarily in her respect for human philosophic thought. However serious and profound that respect is, the consistently growing reverence of the Church for the human person — from the first moment of conception until the last pulse of the brain — is hers because God has gifted her with a deep personal knowledge of a unique person, Jesus Christ. Out of this Faith in Christ, however, the Church hopes always to bring to human thought true light about our beginnings as human persons.

Discussion Questions

1. What are some of the first signs that the new human embryo is organizing itself soon after conception to develop all its eventual body parts?
2. What biological facts indicate that the new human embryo is at the same time organizing itself to one day parent another human embryo?
3. What contribution do these facts make to a person's belief in God?
4. What are some of the main problems in getting Americans today to agree about the beginning of human life?
5. What gives us the signal that a cluster of cells is really an organized body?
6. What kind of knowing and choosing is special to human beings?

Preview of Chapter 8

• Abortion affects an individual human life, not some sort of formless collection of cells.

• Human development during the nine months in the mother's womb is rapid and continuous.

• Abortions are done during all three trimesters (three month periods) of pregnancy. All are violent acts directly attacking the living individual.

• Medical and psychological complications of abortion are numerous, even if not well-publicized.

• There is no absolute medical or psychological reason to abort pregnancy.

• Catholic teaching has always opposed the injustice of destroying unborn human lives. On the Capitol Mall in the shadow of the United States Supreme Court building in Washington, D.C., Pope John Paul II reaffirmed the sacredness of human life from conception on (October 7, 1979).

CHAPTER 8

Abortion in Medicine and Ethics

This chapter will present the medical facts needed to deal intelligently with the moral questions raised by the problem of abortion. In addition, it will examine briefly these moral questions and provide some guidelines.

Abortion is a premature birth before the embryo or fetus can survive outside the mother's womb. Abortions are classified as being either spontaneous or induced. A *spontaneous* abortion, commonly called a miscarriage, occurs because something went wrong with either the placenta or the normal growth of the baby, leading to either premature birth, or the death of the child in the womb. Often it is impossible to determine exactly what went wrong. *Induced* abortion is the willful and forced expulsion of the fetus or embryo from the womb. If the womb in a given case is capable of carrying the child at least to viability, the induced abortion (again, the expulsion of a living fetus prior to viability) is called *elective*. If the womb can in no way do this, and both the mother and the fetal child will die in a short time if the child is not expelled from the womb, the induced abortion can properly be called *therapeutic*, and is not directed intentionally toward fetal death as either an end or a means. *This, it should be noted, is a theological opinion and one that has not been explicitly endorsed by the Magisterium.* Unfortunately, the term "therapeutic" is often used more broadly—and inaccurately—to describe an abortion, induced not to save the mother's life, but for her general well being.

We will consider in this chapter both types of induced abortion. Present abortion technology causes either intrauterine (i.e., in the womb) destruction of the growing child, or causes premature birth with death occurring soon afterwards.

Fetal Development

To understand the medical and biological implications of abortion, it is important to have a knowledge of how the child develops in its mother's uterus (womb). In the embryology text book, *Developmental Anatomy* by Leslie Arey, it is stated: "The formation, maturation and meeting of a female and a male sex cell are all preliminary to their actual union into a combined cell or zygote, which definitely marks the beginning of a new individual."[1] This statement, that an *individual* life starts at fertilization, is true for all species reproducing by sexual reproduction; humans are no exception. Further, when we discuss abortion, it is important to realize that we are concerned with the development and termination of *individual* human lives. We are not discussing evolution, that is, when human life as such first appeared on earth. It must be absolutely clear that we are talking about the growth and development of *individual* human persons.

It is an established biological fact that "like begets like"—chickens always beget chickens, frogs beget frogs, and humans give birth to humans. An embryo always belongs to the same biological species to which its parents belong. This fact is true for the whole biological kingdom—humans are no exception.

We now know from studies in modern genetics that a fertilized egg, as well as all the stages of growth beyond — embryo, fetus, infant, adult — received one-half of its chromosomes (bearers of genes) — the factors which determine inherited characteristics from the male parent, and one-half from the female parent, and keeps them throughout its life. In the early part of their development, many embryos, including human ones, may look like embryos of other species to the naked eye. Nevertheless, they always have the genes and chromosomes of their parents' spe-

---

[1]Leslie Arey, *Developmental Anatomy*, 7th Edition (Philadelphia, W. Saunders and Company, 1974), p. 55.

cies. The old idea that embryos in early development belonged successively to more primitive species, is now known to be wrong. The egg of a human female fertilized by a sperm from a human male is an individual member of the human species from that time of that fertilization, throughout development in the womb of his or her mother, at birth, and throughout life until death overtakes that human person.

The development of the new human individual, as is that of other animals, is rapid and complex, starting from the time of fertilization. Here is a brief timetable describing the various events which take place during growth in the uterus:

AGE	What takes place
1 day	The union of egg and sperm forms the zygote, the beginning of the new individual. The first cell division of the zygote, the first step in its growth, is completed within 36 hours. By future cell divisions (mitosis) all the cells and tissues of the new individual will arise from the zygote.
4 days	Morula state—special techniques can tell the sex of the new individual at this early stage.
7 to 9 days	Blastocyst stage—embyro reaches cavity of uterus and attaches to the lining of the uterine wall, burying itself in its glands.
2.5 to 4 weeks	Neurula stage—by three weeks the foundation for brain, spinal cord and entire nervous system are established. Blood vessels start forming at 2.5 weeks, the heart a day later. At 3.5 weeks the heart, a simple tube, starts to pulsate. From three weeks, the primitive digestive system and the forerunner of the kidney form.
4.5 weeks	The 3 main parts of the brain are present. Eyes, ears, nasal organs, digestive tract, liver, gall bladder and arm and leg buds are forming.
5 weeks	Embryo is 1/3 inch long, and weighs 1/1000 oz. The early differentiation of the cerebral cortex is seen. Pituitary gland begins to form.
5.5 weeks	All muscle blocks present. Baby may begin to move, but mother does not feel this for another 6 to 10 weeks. The heart begins to subdivide into its 4 chambers.

6 weeks	Embryo is 1/2 inch long. Earliest reflexes can be elicited. Electrocardiogram (EKG) and electroencephalogram (EEG) can be recorded. Fingers, then toes, begin to form. Especially during the first 6 to 8 weeks of embryonic life, the embryo is most vulnerable to the effects of drugs, radiations, infections (particularly viral), noxious substances, (such as alcohol and nicotine), and nutritional deficiencies of the mother.
8 weeks	Embryo is 1.5 inches long and weighs 1/30 oz. The face appears quite human. Heart completes the formation of its 4 chambers. Hands and feet are well-formed and distinctly human. Cerebral cortex begins to acquire typical cells. At the end of 8 weeks all organs, facial features and limb structures have begun to form. Everything is present that will be found in the new-born baby. The fundamental plan of the human body is completely mapped out by the end of the second month. During the remainder of pregnancy the various organs will mature in structure and function.
9 weeks	The growing child is now called a fetus. When the eyelids or palms of the hand are touched, they both respond by closing—this indicates that both nerves and muscles are functioning.
10 weeks	Except for refinements, the brain is much as it will be at birth. If the forehead is touched, the fetus turns the head away.
12 weeks *(3 months)*	Fetus is 3-4 inches crown-rump length, and weighs about 1/2 oz. The thumb can now be opposed to the forefinger (a characteristic of all the primates). Fetuses of this age begin to show individual variations, probably based on behavioral patterns from the parents. By the end of the 12th week, the fetus has developed all organ systems and is virtually a functioning organism. The fetal organs become more and more like what they will be in the newborn infant. Dr. Arnold Gessell, in his book *The Embryology of Behavior: The Beginnings of the Human Mind*[2] has writ-

---

[2]New York: Harper, 1945.

ten: "And so, by the close of the first trimester, the fetus is a sentient, moving being. We need not pause to speculate as to the nature of his psychic attributes, but we may assert that the organization of his psychosomatic self is well under way."

4 *months*
Fingerprints, unique to the individual, are formed. The fetus responds to touch, and spontaneously stretches and exercises both arms and legs.

5 *months*
Fetus measures 8 inches crown-rump length, and weighs 8 to 10 oz. The fetus exhibits a firm hand grip, good muscular strength, coordination and reflex action, and kicks, moves, turns in the womb, hiccoughs, develops patterns of sleep and wakefulness, and reacts in an individual way to loud noise, or music or jarring or tapping the abdomen.

6 *months*
During this month, the eyes become sensitive to varying intensities of light and darkness but not to objects.

7 *months*
Fetus measures 12 inches crown-rump length and weighs 2 to 3 pounds. The fetus (now called a premature baby if born) continues growing and maturing. From the 7th to the 9th month, every added day spent in the womb until birth prepares the baby all the better to assume an independent role.

In summary, biological science has shown that:

1) an individual human life begins at fertilization
2) development of the new individual is rapid and continuous throughout life within the womb as well as outside of it.
3) at all times during the individual's development he or she is without any doubt a member of the human species.

Description of Abortion Procedures

A brief description of what is involved in the various abortion procedures is necessary. A human full-term pregnancy is arbitrarily divided into 3 trimesters, each lasting 3 months. The kind of abortion procedure done depends on the length of time the woman has been pregnant. Accordingly, from this perspective there are three classes of abortion.

First trimester abortions. The procedures done during this time are the "dilation and curettage" (D&C) and "suction curettage" (S & C). In a *D & C procedure*, the patient's cervix (neck of the womb) is dilated by inserting into it progressively larger metal dilators. Once the cervix is sufficiently dilated, the lining of the womb is scraped off with a sharp instrument called a curette. This process removes the placenta, membranes and baby. During the procedure the growing embryo/fetus' body is usually dismembered; recognizable parts of the body can be seen in the tissue removed. The doctor doing the abortion must check the tissue which has been removed to make sure that all the parts of the body infant's body are present. In all abortion procedures to be described, this is an important step, because if parts of the body or placenta are left in the womb, the patient will usually develop an infection, or severe bleeding. If all parts are not found, the doctor must re-scrape the uterus (womb) until they are found. Leaving tissue behind is a common complication of abortion done by any procedure.

The *S & C* abortion is done in a similar way, except that instead of scraping away the uterine lining with a curette, the doctor inserts a tube connected to a suction (vacuum) apparatus and sucks the tissue and fetus into a bottle. Here, too, the material obtained is checked for the presence of fetal parts. As the suction is quite strong, the body of the fetus or embryo is much more fragmented than it is by a D & C abortion. Parenthetically, it should be noted that a "mini-abortion" called a menstrual extraction, is sometimes done if a woman's period is a few days late. This is done in the same way as an S & C. Here there would be no *recognizable* fetal parts, as the embryo would only be 2 to 3 weeks old and less than a third of an inch long. In fact, the woman may not even be pregnant.

Second trimester abortions. The procedures done at this time are instillation abortions and "dilatation and evacuation" (D & E).

In an *instillation abortion*, a needle is inserted into the patient's womb, a measured volume of amniotic fluid (the fluid in which the baby is floating while in the womb) is removed, and a solution of prostaglandins (hormone-life substance) or hypertonic (concentrated) salt solution is injected into the womb. *Prostaglandins* cause the uterus to contract, and force the growing fetus to leave the womb prematurely, usually before it can survive outside the womb. Many prostaglandin-aborted infants are born alive, but usually die shortly after birth because of immaturity, particularly of the lungs.

The *hypertonic saline* make the womb contract, and in addition, chemically scalds the baby's delicate skin, causing severe burns. It also causes marked salt imbalance in the fetus, because the salt is swallowed as well as absorbed through the skin. These two effects, salt imbalance and severe burns, usually cause the death of the growing baby before it is actually expelled from the uterus, although occasionally a baby is born alive. In fact, at least two have been known to survive and live to be adopted. Some observers feel the baby suffers pain during the saline procedure, as witnessed by increased fetal movements and heart rate which does not usually occur during prostaglandin abortions. Fetuses *spontaneously* aborted in the second trimester are known to react to painful stimuli when studied outside the womb. Fetuses still in the womb are known to react to unpleasant stimuli, such as needle punctures and sour solutions put into the amniotic fluid.

The D & E abortion is similar to the D & C procedure. The cervix is dilated with either metal dilators, or, the day before the procedure, with the dried stems of the seaweed species *Laminaria* which have been found to cause cervical dilatation. As many of these seaweed stems as possible are inserted into the cervix using dilators, and are allowed to remain overnight. On the day of the abortion procedure using either method of dilation, the uterus is cleaned out by using a specially-designed "ovum forceps," an instrument which can remove placenta, membranes and fetus from the uterus. As before, the fetal body is broken by crushing it with the forceps to allow it to be removed without damaging the cervix. Again, the doctor must make sure that all parts of the fetus' body and the placenta and membranes have been removed.

Third trimester abortions. Instillation abortions can be done during this period. Usually a hysterotomy, an abdominal operation using the same surgical techniques as doing a cesarean section, is performed during this period. Obviously, no effort is made to start the child breathing, as is done during a cesarean delivery. This procedure is usually resorted to when the baby is too big to remove vaginally by a D & E, or when instillation abortions fail. These babies are usually born alive—many will start to breathe on their own but usually die from insufficient development although here also an occasional child survives.

Complications of Induced Abortions

Medical side-effects. There were 1,157,776 legal abortions reported to have been performed in 1978, the latest year for which complete figures are available. In spite of the liberalized abortion laws in this country, illegal (criminal) abortions still occur. When these illegal abortions are performed by non-medically trained persons (including by the pregnant woman herself), the woman undergoing such an abortion is at great risk of losing her life, or developing serious but non-lethal side effects. Accumulated experience is making it obvious that legal abortions also have risks, though to a lesser degree. Clearly, legal abortions are not totally safe procedures.

Death of the mother from abortion, both legal and criminal, can occur. The cause of death is usually hemorrhage and/or infection associated with perforation of the uterus which is a common occurrence. In 1978, 11 women died from legal abortions, and 7 from criminal ones. Contrary to what abortion proponents claimed, legal abortion has *not* put an end to criminal abortions. The figure given here for deaths from legal abortions is the minimum *estimate*.

The Center for Disease Control (CDC), the governmental agency responsible for gathering statistical data on abortions, states in its 1978 report that there is probably under-reporting of legal abortion-related deaths, especially after 1975. Another important point to note is that the CDC in the same report stated that a study they conducted showed that cut-backs in Federal funds for abortions for the poor has *not* resulted in an increase in the number of criminal abortions.

To determine with any degree of accuracy the overall rate of non-lethal side-effects suffered by women who have undergone abortions, whether legal or illegal, is difficult. The CDC reports that about 10% of the women suffer some kind of complication, with 1% suffering a serious complication. Reports in the medical literature by physicians who treat women who were aborted by others suggest that the rates are higher. The reported side effects include prolonged bleeding (sometimes requiring transfusion), severe infection such as peritonitis (inflammation of the lining of the abdominal cavity) with abscess formation, perforation of the uterus, pelvic pain, and urinary tract problems. Occasionally an abdominal operation is necessary to repair uterine or intestinal perforations which occurred during the abortion procedure.

The above are *short-term* complications, usually developing within days or a few weeks after the abortion procedure. What is slowly coming to light is that *legal* abortions also have *long-term* medical complications, especially if the woman has had more than one abortion. These complications include failure to carry subsequent pregnancies to term(Miscarriages and premature births) and infertility. Thus, a woman who has had abortions may find that when finally she wants to have a child, she may either not be able to get pregnant at all or if she does get pregnant, she may not be able to carry the child to term.

Psychological complications. The prevalence of psychological complications is also hard to determine, but it is accepted that such complications indeed occur. These complications are both long-term and short-term and include recurrent anxiety reactions, severe guilt feelings, and depression. Often these problems are intensified at the time of the anniversary of the abortion.

Psychological Effects of Abortion on the Medical Staff

It is becoming recognized that the performance of abortions, especially second trimester ones where body parts of the baby are readily recognizable, are causing psychological effects on the medical staff involved. Articles are appearing in the medical literature describing serious emotional reactions producing physical symptoms in abortion clinic staff persons. These reactions include sleep disturbances, nightmares, effects on interpersonal relationships including increases in the divorce rate, and "moral anguish." The involved medical staff are recognizing the abortion procedure as destructive and violent. This recognition was eloquently stated in a paper presented at a scientific meeting:

> *Those capable of performing or assisting with the procedure [D&E] are having strong personal reservations about participating in an operation which they view as destructive and violent. The same people who cannot help with the procedure applaud its introduction because of increased safety for the patient. Some part of our cultural and perhaps even biological heritage recoils at a destructive operation on a form that is similar to our own, even while we may know that the act has a positive effect for a living person. No one who has not performed this procedure can know what it is like or what it means; but having performed it, we are bewildered by the possibilities of interpretation. We have reached a point in this particular technology where there is no possibility of denial of an act of destruction by the operator. It is before one's eyes. The sensations of dismemberment flow through the forceps like an electric current. It is the crucible of a raging controversy, the confrontation of a modern existential dilemma. The more we seem to solve the problem, the more intractable it becomes.*

Today, is an Abortion Ever Necessary?

Due to modern medical advances, there are hardly any medical conditions in which abortion is absolutely recommended. There can be, it is true, cases in which, if the pregnancy is not terminated forthwith, both mother and non-viable child will shortly perish. Such a diagnosis, of course, must be certain in the judgement of competent medical authority. A second opinion is urged. As instances, many physicians cite cases of septic uterus and of eclampsia badly managed medically and, as a result, finally out-of-control (a predisposition to eclampsia can be detected early in pregnancy by a competent physician and treated so that any threat to the mother or fetal child can be warded off). In these

91

instances an expulsion from the womb which does not involve an attack directed against the fetal child's body can be justified morally within a pro-life context and by the principle of double effect. It may be indeed that in a given case, it is medically certain that continued intrauterine life support will be useless for bringing the fetal child even to viability. For there is no moral obligation to continue a *useless* life-support effort, even if it is the natural uterine one, especially if the price for doing so is the mother's death. Relief from continuing such a futile effort, together with saving the mother's life, is what is both sought and alone intended. The fetus' death, as a result of such an expulsion, is merely tolerated as a secondary effect, because once we have disconnected it from uterine life support, we are, at this stage of medical history, technologically helpless to keep it alive outside.[3]

Pregnant patients with severe kidney disease, lung disease, diabetes and many forms of cancer can be safely carried to term. Even patients with heart disease can be maintained through pregnancy. Current experience has shown that patients with heart failure in the first trimester of pregnancy can survive the added cardiovascular burdens of pregnancy. Some physicians would prefer to abort patients who show heart failure early in pregnancy, but even here it is admitted that most of these patients can be safely carried to term. Pre-existing high blood pressure will not be aggravated by pregnancy. Some physicians suggest that abortion be considered in the condition called "essential hypertention" when changes in the retina of the eye and serious kidney involvement or heart enlargement are present. Here, also, the recommendation is not absolute; even patients who have had a heart attack can survive pregnancy.

In a few rare conditions, the necessity for abortion may appear stronger, but again that necessity is not absolute. Patients who have pheochromocytoma (a tumor secreting adrenal-like hormones), must have their tumor removed surgically, whether or not they are pregnant. The recommended course of treatment is that when the baby is viable, a cesarean section be first performed, and the tumor then is removed afterwards as soon as possible. In a pre-viable child, the tumor is removed, disturbing the uterus as little as possible. It has been found that the mother gains nothing from having the baby aborted. In primary pulmonary hypertension, it is strongly suggested that the patient not get pregnant.

In certain conditions, such as operations to treat cancer of the uterus or cervix discovered during pregnancy or a ruptured tube in

---

[3]M. Zalba, "El aborto terapeutico, aborto indirecto?", in *Estudios eclesiasticos*, 52, (1977), pp. 265–313. Zalba is one of the most eminent theologian consultants working in Rome for the past twenty years for Catholic doctrinal authorities there.

ectopic pregnancy, the child in the diseased uterus or tube is removed with the defective organ. If the child is per chance viable, an attempt is made to deliver it alive. Most often, especially in the case of ruptured tubal pregnancies, the child has already died.

Recently, some physicians have been advocating the removal ("shelling out") of an embryo in a tubal pregnancy long before the tube has begun to break down. They believe that the woman's fertility has a better chance of surviving than if the affected section of the tube is removed (along with the still non-viable fetus) only later in the pregnancy when such removal can no longer be postponed without endangering the mother's life. Obstetrical opinion is divided on this issue, however, many physicians claiming that more scientific and clinical data is needed. A moral evaluation of the procedure must await such data.[4]

It should be emphasized that patients with the rather rare conditions listed above are at somewhat higher risk for developing complications during pregnancy than are otherwise healthy women. They need good medical care during their pregnancy. In addition, it is now recognized by physicians that pregnancy does not cause as serious a burden on the body during disease as once thought. So, it would seem that the vast majority of women, even those afflicted with serious diseases, can survive pregnancy. However, it may be more prudent in some conditions not to get pregnant. Here the woman and her husband must exercise their sexuality in a responsible way.

Psychiatric indications are also not absolute. It has been found that many women who have a genuine psychiatric handicap are more likely to *suffer from abortion* than benefit from one. It has also been found that the prognosis (forecast of outcome) for a post-abortion psychosis is worse than that for a psychosis after childbirth in women with a history of psychiatric problems. There is no indication that pregnant women commit suicide in greater numbers than non-pregnant women, whether they have psychiatric problems or not. There is no evidence that unmarried motherhood leads to any more problems than married motherhood. It seems to be the general opinion that there are no firm psychiatric grounds for terminating a pregnancy.

More recently, many practitioners of in vitro fertilization have deliberately created new situations in which they resort to abortions, even multiple ones in the same pregnancy. For in vitro techniques, as used currently, often involve implanting in the womb four, five, or more living embryos. Practitioners are generally not willing to risk the difficul-

---

[4]Donald McCarthy, "Physicians' Reactions in Ectopic Pregnancy Survey", *Ethics and Medics*, May 1984, and "Ethicists' Reactions to Ectopic Pregnancy Survey, Ibid., September, 1984.

ties which this creates for a successful delivery. Thus, after several weeks, the embryos least-advantageously placed within the womb are deliberately killed by suction tube or by a lethal injection into their developing bodies. Only the one, or at most two, most-promising embryonic children are allowed to continue to term. Here, however, the attack is directed against the bodies of innocent human beings, and in no way can be morally justified.[5]

To summarize with 3 quotations from physicians:

1) "Whatever indications we may use, therapeutic abortion always constitutes a failure of medical science".
2) "In the case of medical indications for abortion, it is possible almost always to give ideal care and avoid the abortion";
3) "There is little evidence that pregnancy in itself worsens a psychosis, either intensifying it, or rendering prognosis for full recovery less likely."

The "Hard Cases," Rape, Incest, Genetic Defect

Rape and incest are truly tragic events in the life of a woman, young or old. Fortunately, the rate of pregnancy in each is low. In rape especially, the threat of contracting venereal disease or of having physical trauma to the reproductive organs is much greater than the threat of pregnancy. It is important to stress that women of all ages, who have been subject to sexual assault, should be seen by a gynecologist as soon as possible for prevention of venereal disease, spermicidal douching, and surgical repair if necessary.

If given from day-2 to day-8 of a woman's cycle, it seems that estrogen or, better, a *low dose* combination of oral contraceptives can prevent
ovulation after a rape attack and, thus, avoid conception. It is still, scientifically unclear whether certain other drugs (dNG, GnRh antagonists, high dosage estrogens and progesterins) have this effect. Research needs to be done also, on other possible non-abortive techniques.[6]

We are not aware of any report in the literature of any severe psychological damage resulting from having to carry a pregnancy resulting from rape to term. In fact, the rape victim is often reported to feel guilt about killing the child.

---

[5]Richard Berkowitz, M.D., *et al.*, "Selective Reduction of Multifetal Pregnancies in the First Trimester", in *The New England Journal of Medicine*, April 21, 1988, pp. 1043–1047.

[6]Lloyd Hess, "Treatment of Rape Victims in Catholic Health Facilities", in *Ethics and Medics*, November and December 1985 and January 1986.

It has also been shown that even very young girls can be carried safely through pregnancy, if they receive good routine prenatal care and supportive counseling. There seems to be a greater need for cesarean delivery, because of their immature bone structure, but there is no indication that pregnancy in any way disproportionately endangers their life, or future reproductive abilities.

No genetic disease in the fetus would endanger the life of the mother. In some cases of conjoint (Siamese) twins, cesarean delivery would be necessary.

There have been reports in the literature of psychiatric problems in women who have aborted defective children. It is important to remember that genetic disease in no way removes the genetically defective child from being a member of the human species; he or she still possesses human chromosomes. Although an individual may perhaps have one more chromosome (trisomy 21) or may be missing part of one (such as in the *cri-du-chat* syndrome), these defects do not remove him/her from membership in the human species.

Summary of the Medical Facts

The data presented in this chapter indicate that the offspring conceived by a human male and a human female is a member of the human species from the time of fertilization throughout its life, even if he/she happens to be born with a genetic defect. Pregnancy is not a disease; even seriously ill women can get pregnant and deliver normal infants. There is no absolute medical or psychological reason to abort a pregnancy, except in cases where it is' morally certain that otherwise both mother and non-viable embryonic or fetal child will shortly die from some pathological condition. In fact, abortions can have serious medical and psychiatric side effects.

Ethical Considerations

These facts have grave moral implications for persons who respect the inviolability of innocent human lives. Since we value human life, then the life of every member of the human species is to be respected; we cannot pick and choose which members of the species we will consider worthy of value. All human individuals have an intrinsic worth and dignity. Consequently, our moral responsibilities in this matter pertains to two areas of human generation: 1) the responsible procreation of new human life, and 2) the preservation of human life once conceived.

Regarding the responsible procreation of new human life, what is critically necessary is the mature use of sexuality, not promiscuity or the use of sexual intercourse merely as a sign of casual friendship. God in His goodness endowed the act of sexual intercourse with pleasure. Indeed, that deep and intimate sharing can also carry with it a great joy. For these reasons, sexual intercourse not only reflects, but also strengthens the bond of love between husband and wife, and enables them to carry more readily the responsibility of parenthood.

Consequently persons who both value human life from its beginning and respect the sexual morality commanded in the sacred scriptures and taught by the church will seek to live a sexually responsible life and not trivialize the acts by which new human life is engendered.

With respect to the preservation of human life once conceived, persons who respect life will be especially vigilant not to destroy a new human life. As discussed in chapter 4, the life of an existing human person is inviolable no matter at what stage of development he or she might be. The Church has over the many centuries protected the life of the unborn. In recent years she has been no less vocal.

The Second Vatican Council was an occasion for the Church to reiterate, and update where necessary, many basic pastoral teachings. In the *Pastoral Constitution on the Church in the Modern World*, the Council Fathers stated simply and forcefully:

> Life must be protected with the utmost care from the moment of conception: abortion and infanticide are abominable crimes.[7]

Nine years later (November 18, 1974), the Vatican Congregation for the Doctrine of the Faith issues another strong affirmation of the Church's traditional teaching on abortion:

> The tradition of the Church has always held that human life must be protected and favored from the beginning, just as at the various stages of its development . . . In the *Didache* [written about 90 A.D.] it is clearly stated: "You shall not kill by abortion the fruit of your womb and you shall not murder the infant already born."[8]

The present Holy Father, Pope John Paul II, has been no less eloquent in his condemnations of abortion. Speaking to 175,000 per-

---

[7]*Gaudium et Spes*, # 5.

[8]Sacred Congregation for the Doctrine of the Faith, Declaration on Abortion (Washington, D.C., USCC Publications, 1975) #6.

sons on October 7, 1979, at the Capitol Mall in Washington, DC he proclaimed:

> I do not hesitate to proclaim before you and before the world that all human life—from the moment of conception and through all subsequent states—is sacred, because human life is created in the image and likeness of God.
>
> All human beings ought to value every person for his or her uniqueness as a creature of God, called to be a brother or sister of Christ by reason of the incarnation and the universal redemption. For us, the sacredness of human life is based on these premises. And it is on these same premises that there is based our celebration of life—all human life. This explains our efforts to defend human life against every influence or action that threatens or weakens it, as well as our endeavors to make every life more human in all its aspects.
>
> And so, we will stand up every time that human life is threatened.
>
> When the sacredness of life before birth is attacked, we will stand up and proclaim that no one ever has the authority to destroy unborn life.[9]

There can be no question that the Church's teaching, current and past, is clear on the issue of abortion. No reason—medical, economic or social—can morally justify a deliberate and direct attack on the life of an innocent human being regardless of age, mental or physical condition, or social status.

Discussion Questions

1. How many significant points can you recall from the nine month development of the unborn child?
2. What are the two kinds of instillation abortions?
3. Why should we expect harmful medical and psychological side effects from abortions?

---

[9]Pope John Paul II, "Stand up for Human Life", *Origins*, Oct. 16, 1979, vol. 9: no. 18, pp 278–280.

4. What are some of the medical conditions of the pregnant mother where abortion is sometimes proposed?
5. What moral responsibility precedes the moral responsibility to preserve human life in the womb?
6. Why is the *Didache* mentioned at the end of this chapter?

Preview of Chapter 9

- The law has not remained neutral about abortion. it actually became more protective of the unborn child as medical knowledge of embryology improved.

- English common law protected the "quickened" fetus as a being with its own right to life.

- State statutes in the United States against abortion were passed in all the states and they gradually eliminated the reference to "after quickening."

- In 1920 Russia legalized abortion, and in 1959 the American Law Institute published a model abortion statute including "Justifiable Abortion."

- The tide had turned against the states liberalizing their abortion laws by late 1972.

- The United States Supreme Court decisions of January 22, 1973, rendered all state statutes against abortion obsolete.

CHAPTER 9

The Law and Abortion

Introduction

What should the law do about abortion? Can this procedure be treated like any other medical procedure? If so, the law might be content to punish medical negligence and to insist on licensed practitioners of abortion. The law could also protect a pregnant woman's right to have an adequate medical explanation of the abortion procedure and to give informed consent before it took place. The law would regulate abortion as it regulates other medical procedures.

But abortion is not just another medical procedure. Abortion kills a developing human being while still hidden in the protective environment of the mother's womb. The law punishes killing innocent human beings outside the womb. In fact, the law exists to provide all citizens the opportunity for "life, liberty, and the pursuit of happiness." Can the law remain neutral about killing in the womb?

Actually, *human law has not remained neutral about abortion.* During the 300 years from 1620 to 1920, scientific embryology uncovered in marvelous detail the continuity in development and the new individual identity of each human being from fertilization of the ovum through the birth event. And human laws became correspondingly more protective of those tiny unborn members of the human family.

These laws reflected medical data and the political theory of civil rights. Since 1920, the year of the initial Russian legalization of abortion under Lenin, laws against abortion around the world have undergone considerable compromise in their protection of the unborn. Social concerns like population growth and family planning for the poor are listed as reasons for abortion. Increased sensitivity to the burden of pregnancy for unmarried mothers and to the shock of unplanned pregnancy for married mothers now supports the slogan, "a woman's right to choose an abortion."

In the conclusion of chapter 5 of this *Handbook*, the legal acceptance of abortion is included in the designation of a "pro-death ideology." On the other hand, when the law protects the lives of the unborn, the defective, and the comatose, it manifests a "pro-life ideology." In the case of both pro-death and pro-life ideologies, the law reflects moral judgments about human life. Through the contemporary trend to legalize abortion, the generally pro-life ideology of law is matched with the pro-death ideology of abortion. This has necessitated drawing a line at the rather arbitrary moment of human birth to divide two ideologies.

Notice two implications of this mixture of ideologies. First, the line drawn at birth can easily be drawn again at the onset of irreversible coma, which would legalize mercy killing. Secondly, the pro-death ideology of abortion does not simply imply neutrality about abortion to honor a pregnant woman's private conscience and personal morality. The ideology itself goes a step farther—it withdraws the civil rights and legally protected existence of the entire class of unborn human beings. *Abortion of human lives necessarily remains a matter of public morality, but now it becomes a morality of public approval.* This chapter will review the law and abortion, culminating with the current situation in the United States.

Historical Overview

The practice of abortion did not begin with modern medicine. It apparently existed in more primitive forms throughout recorded history. Even without benefit of extensive modern knowledge about human development in the womb, the ancient Code of Hammurabi, when promulgated about 1728 B.C., contained prohibitions against abortion. In the 12th century B.C., the Assyrian King Tiglath-Pileser I codified certain laws including prohibitions against abortion.

Anthropological studies of primitive societies reveal in one form or another a sense that abortion violates the sacred and brings punishment. *The Old Testament of the Bible does not discuss induced abortion but this merely indicates that the Israelite view of children as a gift of God made legislation against abortion unnecessary.*

Yet ancient pagan cultures also tolerated abortion in various ways. Roman law did not take a firm stand against abortion until Septimus Severus (193-211 A.D.), a reform emperor, treated abortion as an "extraordinary crime" with no definite penalty, although he decreed exile for the wife practicing abortion.

The emerging European nations tended to model their civil law on the cannon law of the Church. As early as the sixth century A.D., the law of the Visigoths provided a death penalty for anyone who gave a potion to cause an abortion. Anglo-Saxon law before the Norman conquest of 1066 provided both civil and ecclesiastical penalties for abortion. Henry De Braxton, who administered the king's law in the mid-thirteenth century, included a provision considering abortion to be homicide if the fetus were formed or animated.

In England, Sir Edward Coke, a noted scholar of the common law, wrote in 1650 that to cause a woman to deliver a dead child was not murder but a "misprision." This latter term meant a criminal act closely related to a capital crime. If the aborted child were born alive and then died as a result of the abortion, the crime was murder.

A century later, William Blackstone, in his famous *Commentaries on the Law*, wrote that "Life is the immediate gift of God, a right inherent by nature in every individual; and it begins in contemplation of law as soon as an infant is able to stir in the mother's womb"[1] This statement clearly gives legal protection from the point of "quickening" when the mother can feel movement in her womb. Thus the common law of England protected the "quickened" fetus as a being with its own right to life, immune from destruction at the mother's will.[2] Whether induced abortion before quickening was a criminal act in common law has been disputed.

In 1803, the first British statute against abortion condemned as a felony any attempt to procure an abortion. The act had to be willful, malicious and unlawful, but not necessarily effective or harmful to the mother. If the attempt were made after quickening, the punishment

---

[1]Blackstone, *Commentaries on the Laws of England.* p. 124 (1769)

[2]Means, Cyril, "The Law of New York Concerning Abortion". 14 N.Y.L.F., 411. 508 (1968).

could be death. If before quickening, the punishment could be whipping, imprisonment, or exile to a penal colony for up to 15 years.[3]

Thus this British statute cleared up any confusion in common law about the act of abortion before quickening—it, too, was a felony, although the penalty was reduced. This clear legal protection of the human fetus before quickening, which occurs in the 12th to 16th week of pregnancy, preceded much of the modern embryological research which shows the marvelous continuity of fetal development. This first British abortion law strongly influenced the individual states of the new United States of America in their abortion legislation.

United States Law on Abortion

British common law on abortion was generally followed in the 13 original states before and after the Declaration of Independence. But gradually each state passed its own statutes. The earlier statutes were usually severe with abortion after quickening, but lenient or silent concerning abortion before that event. This was the common law tradition. But gradually the distinction on quickening was removed, so that in 1965 that distinction differentiated the abortion penalty in only 10 states.[4] Thus the British statute of 1803 and its 1837 amendment, which had eliminated all references to quickening, seemed to give examples to the states in their legislation.

In fact, emerging scientific evidence was proving that quickening could not represent a difference between human life and non-life. Already in 1823 a standard American work on medical law by Theodoric and John Beck argued for "vitality" from the moment of conception on grounds of reason and physiology. They concluded:

> If physiology and reason justify the position just laid down, we must consider those laws which treat with less severity the crime of producing abortion at an early period of gestation, as immoral and unjust.[5]

Most early state statutes made no reference to therapeutic abortion or abortion to save the life of the mother. However, in the course of time 46 states and the District of Columbia incorporated such a qualification

---

[3]Grisez, Germain G., *Abortion. the Myths. the Realities. and the Arguments.* (N.Y.,Corpus Books, 1970), p. 188.

[4]*Ibid.*, p. 191.

[5]*Elements of Medical Jurisprudence, Vol. 1* (Albany, 1823),202–203. 203.

in their statutes. Only Louisiana, Pennsylvania, New Jersey, and Massachusetts did not, and the latter two states had had judicial decisions which allowed therapeutic abortion.[6]

The genuine legislative concern which prompted these statutes protecting the unborn was seen as a logical expression of the common law tradition. Thus in 1850 the Supreme court of Pennsylvania wrote about the "civil rights" of an infant *en ventre sa mere* (in the mother's womb), saying they are fully protected at all periods after conception.[7] The unborn were accorded property rights, and by the time of the Second World War courts were even according damages for prenatal injuries to infants in the womb. The dean of authorities on such cases, William Prosser, has maintained that "the unborn child in the path of an automobile is as much a person in the street as the mother."[8]

Two examples of modern judicial decisions in the United States preferring the rights of unborn children over the rights of parents are significant. The New Jersey Supreme court in 1964 ordered a mother to accept blood transfusions contrary to her expressed religious convictions, to save the life of her unborn child.[9] In a 1940 case, a California District Court allowed the guardian of an unborn child to sue for support from the father when the fetus was less than six months old.[10]

The picture drawn thus far of legal protection of the unborn seems to reflect an increasing awareness of the scientific reality of fetal development. In the period from 1880 to 1955 science was unlocking the secrets of the cell's chromosomal patterns with genetic components unique to each human embryo and the molecular structure of DNA, the plasma of life. It was found that a single thread of DNA from a human cell contains personal information equivalent to a library of one thousand volumes, or fifty sets of the *Encyclopedia Britannica*. But social factors were at work to undermine the legal protection of unborn human beings.

Twentieth Century Liberalization of Abortion Laws

One date marking a clear shift in legal protection for the unborn is November 18, 1920. On that date the Commissariats of Health and Justice of the Soviet Union legalized abortion without charge as long as it was done by physicians in hospitals. In 1922 in Moscow hospitals there were

---

[6]Grisez, *op. cit.*. p. 191
[7]*Mills v. Commonwealth of Pennsylvania*, 13 Pa. St. 631 (1850).
[8]*Prosser on Torts*. 3d Edit, 1964, Sec. 56.
[9]42 n. J. 421, 201 A 2d 538 (1964).
[10]38 C. A. 2d 122, 100 P. 2d 806 (1st District 1940).

35,520 births and 7,769 abortions. By 1929 there were 51,059 births and 82,017 abortions. By 1936, a stricter policy attempted to limit abortions for population reasons, but in 1955 a new liberalization was decreed.[11]

Liberalization followed the Soviet precedent in Nazi Germany and the Scandinavian countries. After the Second World War, the Eastern European countries followed the Russian example of liberalization. Western European nations generally restricted abortions to life-saving circumstances for the mother. However, in the 1960s, the worldwide movement toward more permissive abortion laws picked up momentum. It brought about the 1967 Abortion Act of England, Scotland, and Wales. This law permits abortion if pregnancy would involve risk to the life or physical or mental health of the mother, or if there is substantial risk that the child to be born would be seriously handicapped. A so-called "social clause" of the bill also admits abortions for social and economic reasons within the family.

Meanwhile, in the United States, the year 1959 marks a turning point in the movement toward relaxing the anti-abortion laws. In that year the American Law Institute published a tentative draft of a revised statute on abortion to be included in its "Model Penal Code." The model statute would include a category of "Justifiable Abortion" in specific categories of cases. These cases, however, were defined with vague and elastic phrases like "gravely impair the physical or *mental health* of the mother," or, "the child would be born with *grave* physical or *mental defect*".

Unlike the statutes in existence in about half the states, the new proposal did not require that the ground for justifying the abortion be in fact present, *but only that the physician believe it to be so.* To prosecute a physician for unjustifiable abortion one would have to prove that he or she *did not believe* any of the justifying conditions to be fulfilled. The statute appeared rather restrictive at first glance, but actually allowed a very broad area for arbitrary judgment by licensed physicians.

On April 25, 1967, Colorado was the first state to enact an abortion law and modeled after the American Law Institute proposal. Before that happened, at least four legislatures (Illinois, Minnesota, New York, and New Hampshire) had rejected similar statutes. But North Carolina and California followed Colorado in 1967, and ten more states followed suit in the next several years. Then, in 1970, Alaska, Hawaii, New York, and Washington all enacted permissive abortion statutes.

But, after June, 1970, when the New York statute passed, Florida was the only additional state to legalize abortion, while 33 states debated the issue and voted against permitting abortion for any reason except to

---

[11]Grisez, *op.cit..* pp. 194–200.

save the life of the mother. *In two states in 1972 public referenda rejected abortion on demand during the first 20 weeks of pregnancy* (North Dakota by 78% opposition and Michigan by 63% opposition). New York even repealed its law in May, 1972, by larger margins in the State Assembly and Senate than the 1970 bill had in passing. However, Governor Nelson Rockefeller vetoed the repeal bill and the permissive law remained in effect. These facts indicate that the tide had turned against liberalized abortion laws by the end of 1972. But January 22, 1973, became a new date to remember.

The Supreme Court Decisions

The United States supreme Court on January 22, 1973, decided two cases involving abortion, *Roe v. Wade* and *Doe v. Bolton*. In the first case, the court decreed that "the right of personal privacy includes the abortion decision" and that "the word *person* as used in the Fourteenth Amendment doe not include the unborn." In substance, the Court decided that, for the first three months of pregnancy, the abortion decision and its implementation must be left to the medical judgment of the woman's attending physician. Obviously, she may choose as a physician an abortion practitioner. After the first three months the states may regulate the abortion procedure in ways that are reasonably related to maternal health. This would include regulation setting medical standards for such abortions.

Finally, in the stage after viability (the third trimester or three months of pregnancy), the Court decreed that the state may even forbid abortion except where it is necessary for the life or *health of the mother*. The Court interpreted "health" in very broad terms, referring to factors that might include such considerations as "physical, emotional, psychological, familial, the woman's age, distressful life and future, the unwanted child, and unwed motherhood." *The Court throughout the decision refers to the fetus as a form of potential human life.*

The companion case, *Doe v. Bolton*, struck down those parts of the Georgia criminal law on abortion which established a residency requirement; demanded that the abortion be performed in a licensed hospital or clinic in the first trimester; made committee approval necessary; and established the two-doctor concurrence requirement. It declared that a broad concept of the health of the mother may be used to justify the life or health of the unborn child.

The decisions of the Court were rendered by seven justices in favor, with justices White and Rehnquist dissenting. In the *Roe v. Wade* case

106

the decision stated that it is doubtful "that abortion was ever firmly established as a common law crime even with respect to the destruction of a quick fetus." In the light of the common law tradition that has already been discussed in this chapter—the Supreme Court statement seems ill-founded and incorrect.[12] The Supreme Court also argued that the few state courts called upon to interpret their abortion laws in the late 19th and 20th centuries focused on protecting the mother's health rather than in preserving the embryo and fetus. But at least 11 state decisions had clearly said that protection of the life of the unborn child was at least one of the purposes of their state statutes, and 9 other decisions imply the same intent. Only 4 decisions can be cited supporting the Supreme Court interpretation.[13] In any case, after the 1973 decisions of the Supreme Court, the various state statutes prohibiting abortion became obsolete.

The essential legal position of the majority opinion of the Supreme Court states that "the unborn have never been recognized in the law as persons in the whole sense." The pro-life movement in the United States quickly pointed out the parallel to the March 6, 1857, Dred Scott decision of the Supreme Court which ruled that black persons were not "legal" persons according to the United States Constitution. Eleven years and a civil war later, that mistake was corrected by the 13th and 14th amendments to the Constitution.

Opponents of the Supreme Court decisions of 1973 are calling for a Human Life Amendment to the United States Constitution. The United States Catholic Bishops reacted quickly to the January 22, 1973 decisions. On February 13, 1973, they described the decisions as "erroneous, unjust, and immoral," and, "entirely contrary to the fundamental principles of morality."

Leaders in the pro-life movement sought to provide whatever legal restraints were feasible. One highly successful effort promoted "conscience clauses" so that individuals and institutions would not be forced to perform or participate in abortions. The Court had only ruled that states could not punish persons for performing abortions in certain circumstances, but it was clear that efforts would now be made to compel physicians or hospitals to perform abortions or at least cut them off form public funds if they did not do so. *Within a year after the January 22, 1973, decisions, 17 states and the Federal government had enacted legislation establishing conscience clauses.*

---

[12]See "Abortion and the Supreme Court", in *Abortion and Social Justice.* edited by T. W. Hilgers and D. J. Horan, (New York, Sheed & Ward, 1972), Epilogue, pp. 301–322,esp. pp. 311–312.

[13]*Ibid..* p. 312.

However, state legislation to control abortion could accomplish little. On July 1, 1976, in *Planned Parenthood v. Danforth*, the Supreme Court struck down a Missouri statute requiring that a husband give his consent before his wife could undergo a first trimester abortion. It also ruled out the requirement that an unmarried girl under the age of 18 have the consent of a parent in a first trimester abortion. This decision weakened the Court's support for the intimacy and unity of the marital relationship and undermined the rights of parents to direct the upbringing of their own children.

Three decisions the next year, on June 20, 1977, marked a reversal of the Court's trend of liberalization. The Supreme Court ruled in *Maher v. Roe* and *Poelker v. Doe* that it is not unconstitutional to exclude non-therapeutic abortion from municipal hospitals and state medical assistance programs, while at the same time these services and benefits are extended to childbirth. In *Beale v. Doe* the Court upheld a Pennsylvania law limiting Medicaid assistance to those abortions certified by physicians as medically necessary.

Numerous other abortion-related decisions of the Supreme Court have extended the applications of the above cases. The most noteworthy is *Harris v. McRae* of June 30, 1980, which ruled constitutional the Hyde Amendment, legislation which limits the use of Medicaid funds to pay for abortions.

Subsequent Developments

Efforts to restrict the actual performance of abortions have been vigorously supported since 1973 by outstanding political leaders and a broad-based pro-life movement.

Two major initiatives of the pro-life forces seeking to restrict abortions were launched in 1981. On January 19, 1981, Senator Jesse Helms introduced in the Senate a human life statute that declared a fetus is a human being from the moment of conception. A second initiative of 1981 occurred on September 21st, when Senator Orrin Hatch introduced a constitutional amendment declaring that a right to abortion is not secured by the Constitution and that Congress and the several States should have concurrent power to restrict and prohibit abortion.

However, the most important development to date has been a Supreme Court decision issued on July 3, 1989, concerning a Missouri State law which restricted abortion. The Missouri statute had declared that "the life of each human being begins at conception" and "unborn children have protectable interests in life, health, and well-being" (Preamble to the Missouri law); that a physician prior to performing an abortion on a woman whom he believes is 20 or more weeks pregnant, must test to see if the fetus is viable; that the use of public employees and facilities to perform or assist abortions was prohibited, except when necessary to save the mother's life; and that it was unlawful to use public funds, employees or facilities to counsel or encourage a woman to have an abortion not necessary to save her life. A United States Court of Appeals had ruled that these provisions violated Roe v. Wade.

The U.S. Supreme Court said that the statements of the Preamble to the Missouri statute should not be invalidated; that the prescriptions concerning testing for viability and the restrictions concerning the use of public funds, employees, and facilities are *not* in conflict with Roe V. Wade or other Supreme Court decisions. A state may favor childbirth over abortion.

Future prospects of legal control of abortion depend most heavily on continuing sensitizing of both opinion-makers and the general public to the social injustice of abortion. Simultaneous efforts at achieving social justice for the poor and the elderly and all other victims of discrimination will lend credibility and success to the cause of unborn human beings.

Discussion Questions

1. Can you review the development of British common law and later British statutes on abortion?
2. Can you review the development of United States statutes on abortion up to 1972?
3. What indications are there that the tide had turned against liberalizing state abortion laws in the United States by late 1972?
4. What did the two United States Supreme Court decisions of January 22, 1973, say about abortions in the three trimesters of pregnancy?
5. What did the Supreme Court decisions of 1977 and 1989 do about abortion?

PART THREE

Critical Issues in Caring for Human Life

Preview of Chapter 10

- The patient's rights come from his responsibilities as a person.

- The patient has responsibility for the intelligent use of freedom.

- The patient has a right to help from others in cultivating his intelligent use of freedom.

- From his fundamental obligation as a person flow the patient's responsibility and right:

- to give consent based on accurate information

- to maintain life.

- to recover from illness.

- to choose a physician.

- to cultivate a healthy life-style.

- to maintain privacy as to personal matters.

- to treat others maturely.

CHAPTER 10

A Patient's Responsibilities and Rights

As this chapter on the *rights* of patients was being planned, it was recognized that it would have to speak also to the responsibilities of patients. *For human rights flow from human responsibilities.* And responsibilities flow from the call God gives to each of us to be and to act as human beings. As a matter of fact, the very word "responsibility" means a *response* which is required of us because of that *call.*

This call is not made up of mere words; it comes from the way God made us. It begins at the moment of conception.

Our responsibilities and rights which flow from them, then, came from our first moments as human *persons.* To be a person means to have the need and capacity for *intelligent freedom.* We have this need and capacity from the first moment of our existence, regardless of whether we are at any given moment actually exercising the intelligent freedom to which we are called. Thus from the moment of conception to the moment of death and all the days in between each of us experiences, as persons, a life lived in intelligent freedom.

Called to Love Self and Others

In the early 1960's a number of writers won themselves a large reading public by selling a radical individualism. They trumpeted their cause: Every person for himself, and let no government or other power ask anyone to sacrifice himself for others.

While full of anti-Christian exaggerations, this radical individualism nonetheless has something to teach us about being a person: *To seek one's own genuine self-fulfillment is not sinful.* Indeed the Christian would see this as a duty, for it amounts to using the gifts God has given us. Intelligent freedom means, first of all, taking charge of *one's own life.* While the individualists are correct in championing the need for this internal "self-possession," the goal a person must have in his intelligent use of freedom must include also a project of building a life *outside* himself. The only project outside the person truly worthy of him as a person is the building up of a community of persons of which he is a member. There is a need to build family, friendships, and a society.

These communities of persons are necessary if we are to be born and survive. None of us can have access all alone to all we need materially, beginning from the body which two other beings supplied us. It is an understatement to say that a community of persons is a very useful instrument for one's individual survival.

But it would be a serious mistake to look on this humanly necessary community of persons as simply a useful tool. For, as much as material necessities, we need to share in the inner lives of others. We need to communicate our ideals and joys, our worries and sorrows, with them, and they with us. We need their support and esteem, and they ours. This comes only through the sometimes hard, but always deeply satisfying work we call love.

Patients Are Persons, Too

Patients, like all other persons, are *called* by God to *act* like persons. This means: (1) self-possession, or fundamental control over one's own person; and (2) building a genuine community of persons. Patients, like anyone else, must respond to this call; that is, they have a responsibility, and thus a right, to live not as things, but as persons. They have a right to expect respect for themselves, their families, and friends. This respect

114

means that no patient will ever be used simply as a tool for getting what someone else wants. It means reverence for each person, no matter how much his intelligent freedom remains yet undeveloped, or how much of it has been lost to him.

Goal of Health Care: To Help Persons Be Persons

Health care professionals do not confer on the patient the power to get well. That power is already in the person. Hospitals and medical personnel simply help that power to become active and produce health. The purpose of this help is to contribute to what the patient has to do as a person: To be in possession of his own life, and to build his place in a community of persons through love.

It is the medical profession's function, however, only to *help* the patient do this. The primary responsibility and right to reach these goals are the *patient's*, no one else's! The responsibility and right to make intelligent decisions cannot be delegated away to health care professionals or to society at large. Even where a legitimate proxy must speak for a child or for a comatose person, it must always be with the aim of presenting as accurately as possible, under the circumstances, what the *patient* would decide to do, were he able. Nor can the patient make any completely unlimited claims on the resources society has to offer for health care. The goal of health care is always to *help* persons to move towards whatever intelligent freedom is possible to them.

Informed Consent

To exercise freedom intelligently over one's own life and to live in community with other persons, a patient has the responsibility of making a conscientious judgment based on solid information about any proposed treatment. Often treatment will be so simple or routine as not to require much scrutiny. But whether this is so or not must be something the patient judges, no one else.

Even more, the decision to use more drastic forms of therapy may not be left simply in the hands of the physician, "no questions asked". No one has a right, for instance, to continue or discontinue expensive or painful complicated technologies of life support (respirators, stomach tube feeding, or such) *simply* on the basis that: "The doctor said to do it." The health professional has special competence in medicine, not necessarily in ethics. It is wrong for anyone to deliberately fail to seek an informed conscience or to follow it. Deep within his conscience man discovers a law which he has not laid upon himself but which he must obey. Its voice, ever calling him to love and to do what is good and to avoid evil, tells him inwardly at the right moment: do this, shun that. For man has in his heart a law inscribed by God. His dignity lies in observing this law, and by it he will be judged. His conscience is man's most secret core, and his sanctuary. There he is alone with God whose voice echoes in his depths. By conscience, in a wonderful way, that law is made known which is fulfilled in the love of God and of one's neighbor. Through loyalty to conscience Christians are joined to other men in the search for truth and for the right solution to so many moral problems which arise both in the life of individuals and from social relationships. Hence, the more a correct conscience prevails, the more do persons and groups turn aside from blind choice and try to be guided by the objective standards of moral conduct.[1]

This does not mean that a person may not allow a medical procedure for himself unless he is absolutely sure it is the best choice. It means only that he must make the best effort he can to discover the right thing.

> Yet it often happens conscience goes astray through ignorance which it is unable to avoid, without thereby losing its dignity. This cannot be said of a man who takes little trouble to find out what is true and good, or when conscience is by degrees almost blinded through the habit of committing sin.[2]

To form his conscience, the patient has a responsibility and therefore a right to be informed by his physician about what the diagnosis is; what medication, surgery or other intervention the doctor proposes; and how this procedure may affect his life and the course of his disease. This puts upon the patient the responsibility to speak to the physician honestly and frankly. It also gives the patient the right to be listened to carefully and to be believed.

This right to be informed, though real, is not unlimited. It applies mainly to the medical procedure and to its predictable results, though it also applies to informing the patient of his present condition as known through diagnosis. If, however, the physician knew that a particular patient, knowing of his condition, would do unjustified damage to himself, to his chances for recovery, or to someone else, the physician would not be obliged to reveal the diagnosis. This problem could arise with a highly nervous patient who, the physician is sure, would hear the word

---

[1]*Constitution on the Church in the Modern world. (Gaudium et Spes.).* #16.
[2]*Ibid.*

"cancer" and thereupon give up all effort at a cure which is actually quite feasible. Another case might arise where a pregnant woman wants an amniocentesis performed with the declared intention of aborting should there be indications of a defective fetus.

In order to judge what decision should be made on the basis of the information the physician can offer, the patient also has a responsibility to search out worthwhile standards of morality. The patient should know, for example, that there is a tremendous moral difference between allowing death to come naturally through the inner breakdown of one's own body systems, and aiming to bring death on through lethal drugs. He should know that, while one may be justified in not expending great effort to prolong a life of misery and pain, yet one must take reasonable efforts to prolong a life which is going to be merely to some degree and in some way substandard, as in the case of a Down's Syndrome child.

For a Catholic, such standards of morality are rooted in the Church's union with and personal knowledge of Jesus Christ. The implications of the Church's experience of Jesus as a Person, divine and human, for daily Christian living are reflected in the moral positions upheld by her Bishops teaching in union with the Bishop of Rome. From the patient's responsibility to know and judge his life by standards rooted in Jesus Christ comes the right of the patient for an honest and clear moral teaching from priests and other Catholics. Pope John Paul I made this point on the very day of his own untimely death:

> "Among the rights of the faithful, one of the greatest is the right to receive God's word in all its entirety and purity."[3]

Life

The patient has a responsibility to stay alive, and therefore the right to whatever help is necessary from health care professionals to do this. In this maintenance of life against disease which is a present and serious threat to life, the patient is expressing his reverence and gratitude for the gift of life through which God makes it possible for him to experience freedom, intelligence, creativity, and love.

Reverence and gratitude for these gifts was typical of Jesus in his own earthly days, and in this he was showing forth the attitude of his Father towards human life.

---

[3]*Osservatore Romano.* September 29, 1978

Abba (O Father), you have the power to do all things. Take this cup away from me, But let it be as you would have it, not as I. (Mk. 14:36)

The patient who wants to be genuinely Christian must, then, love life, and, like Jesus, tolerate the possibility of its slipping away only as an opportunity to embrace the will of the Father. Death is acceptable, therefore, only as an opportunity to have life restored in a new way in the eventual resurrection of the body alive in the Risen Jesus.

Death, as it is experienced in the Christian view, is the result of sin's entrance into human history.

Therefore just as through one man sine entered the world and with sin death . . . death reigned even over those who had not sinned. . . .(Rm. 5:12–14)

The last enemy to be destroyed is death. (1 Cor. 15:26)

God did not make death, nor does he rejoice in the destination of the living. (Wis. 1:13)

The Christian cannot, therefore, be in love with death. It is misleading, moreover, to speak of a "right to die." What a person does have, of course, when death is showing itself inevitably near, is the right not to have his *dying* dragged out for *no good reason*. Here again it is the responsibility of the patient, and of no one else, to decide whether there are good reasons to slow down the dying process. In making this decision he has a right to know from his physician how costly such an attempt will be in pain, expenses, incapacitation, and the like. Additionally, he has a right to whatever help physicians, hospitals, family, friends and society can afford to give him without impinging on the basic rights of others.

Dedication to maintaining one's own life must come from a deep personal, and responsible decision within the patient as a person. Each of us must, moreover, seek to guide our feelings and our actions into harmony with such a position. Psychiatrists have noted that a number of people who have made "decisions" favoring life yet act in ways that are detrimental to their own well being. Once again, just as there is a patient's responsibility in this area, so also there is a patient's right to be supported by pastors, family, friends, and health care professionals in maintaining this pro-life attitude. If it has deteriorated for some reason, the patient has a right to help in re-building it.

118

Health

Each of us has a responsibility to stay alive. We are called to something further, however: we are called to a good quality of life; that is, to health. Being alive is a start, but not enough. Each of us must make a free and deep commitment to good health. We are responsible to maintain optimal health, to assist in our own recovery of health, and to be rehabilitated when necessary.

This commitment to which we are called gives us the right to be helped in fulfilling it. Jesus illustrated this in his parable of the Good Samaritan who recognized this right in the wounded stranger and

was moved to pity at the sight. He approached him and dressed his wounds, pouring in oil and wine. (Lk. 10:33–34)

The right to be helped belongs to each person because of the basic value each human being has within him. The community does not, for example, bestow on an infant the right to be free from every defect which medicine can prevent or correct. God does that. The community has a moral obligation to recognize that right and actively support it. *Even more, the community has an obligation to protect the individual from any significant risk to his life for the benefit of another, as in the case of experiments for which no valid consent has been given.*

Choosing a Physician

The responsibility and right of pursuing health necessarily implies that of choosing a physician and asking for help. All the professionals in health care, including physicians, have an obligation to offer help to the patient in making such a choice and in encouraging the patient to follow through in seeking help. The patient has a right to know both the competency and ethical integrity of a recommended physician or hospital. For recent studies have turned up alarming figures regarding substandard competency of 30% to 50% among American doctors and hospitals.[4]

---

[4]See studies cited in *Health Care Ethics. A Theological Analysis.* by Benedict M. Ashley, O. P., and Kevin D. O'Rourke, O. P. (St. Louis, MO: The Catholic Health Association, 1982, Second Edition) pp. 73–74.

Life Style

Every individual is called by God to build for himself a life style which recognizes the requirements for good health and pursues them in a practical way. Consumption of medicines and stays in the hospital are no substitutes for simplicity and regularity in daily schedule, control over diet and smoking, and moderation in exercise. Sexual promiscuity and abuse of drugs endanger health as well as destroy one's right appreciation of the place which sexual activity and sophisticated pharmaceuticals can have in one's life.

Privacy

Patients of necessity make themselves vulnerable in relation to the physician, to other health care professionals, and to institutions such as hospitals. They must of necessity in these circumstances make known their physical problems. They will also at times, even though perhaps only indirectly, reveal their personal moral failings or domestic or business difficulties. At the same time, they have the responsibility and right to protect themselves from the misuse of such information.

This right of the patient requires a recognition of his right to privacy on the part of health care professionals. *It is by no means an unlimited right, of course, and every patient must accept this fact when he seeks medical help, even though the limitations have not been spelled out in detail.* For instance, a physician must reveal it to the proper authorities when he discovers that the patient is going to do some serious harm to a third party. Thus, for example, even if the law does not pose a legal obligation, a doctor has a moral obligation to inform the parents of a pregnant teenage girl that their daughter is planning an abortion, if he knows this to be the case.

Such revelations, however, are exceptions to the rule. Any physician's information, hospital records, or computer data regarding a patient must be guarded against any violation of the patient's justified right to privacy.

Maturity

The patient, by reason of his illness, does not lose the responsibility for personal spiritual and emotional maturity in dealing with others. *Spiritual maturity means here ethical maturity: that is, the steadfast refusal to use other persons as mere instruments.*

120

This implies a willingness not to use the facilities and services which health care professionals and hospitals make available in a way which goes against the moral commitments of those persons and institutions. Thus it would be a kind of spiritual immaturity to expect a Catholic hospital to care for a patient who by an unreasonable refusal to eat or take medicine is in effect deliberately committing suicide. The same would be true of a woman seeking amniocentesis testing with the intention, contrary to the moral commitment of a hospital or physician, to obtain an abortion.

The patient also has responsibility to gain insight into and progressive mastery over serious emotional immaturity. Self-hatred can seduce a person into seeking pain or punishment from the hands of unsuspecting medical professionals. Self-pity can feed a craving for attention and care from already overburdened nurses or doctors. Persons whose lives are not filled with the genuine drama of growing personal self-possession or the building of personal relations through authentic love can easily seek substitute drama for their empty lives through sickness, complaining, obscure ailments, medication, or operations.

Finally, patients are called to responsibility towards physicians, nurses, medical technicians, and institutions by following competent advice, cooperating with therapy, respecting feelings, showing gratitude, protecting reputations, and giving fair and prompt payment.

When a patient is violating these responsibilities of emotional and ethical maturity, the victims have a right and in most cases an obligation forcefully to put a stop to it.

Discussion Questions

1. Why do we recognize certain rights of a patient only on the basis of his responsibilities?
2. Why and in what sense is it not selfish for the patient to insist on looking out for himself?
3. Is there anything wrong in a patient's attitude to "doing whatever the doctor says?"
4. Does a patient who is tired of living have a right to seek death?
5. What should a physician do about a patient who ignores all his instructions?
6. What could happen to a person who does not maintain any personal privacy at all?

Preview of Chapter 11

● The most frequently transplanted organ today is the kidney, with about 3,500 transplants each year in the United States.

● Human organs cannot at present be preserved by deep-freezing techniques. Instead, a process of perfusion circulates a special fluid through the blood vessels of the organ.

● Tissue rejection must be controlled for the successful transplantation of an organ.

● Catholic teaching permits organ transplantation from both cadavers and living donors under certain safeguards.

● Living donors may not give an unpaired organ such as the heart, nor an organ necessary for the body's functional integrity (such as an eye).

● In the case of a shortage of organs, the recipients must not be chosen for purely pragmatic reasons of wealth or social worth.

CHAPTER 11

Organ Transplantation Today

Introduction

Probably the majority of people living in nations sharing the western culture have heard about organ transplantation. Organ transplantation involves the removal of an organ from a cadaver or a living human donor and implanting it in a recipient who is in need of it. The most commonly transplanted organs and tissues are kidneys, corneas, hearts, livers, and bone marrow.

The most frequently transplanted organ today is the kidney. While the first successful kidney transplantation was done in 1950, by 1981 over 35,000 successful transplants had been performed in the United States. Currently, there are about 3,500 renal (kidney) transplants done each year and there are approximately 18,000 persons walking around with somebody else's kidney in their bodies. Nonetheless, in the United States alone over 13,000 patients are waiting for kidneys to become available. In the meanwhile, they need chronic hemodialysis (kidney machines) in order to stay alive. The limiting factor in the transplantation of kidneys today apparently is the shortage of donor kidneys. Wide publicity has been given to the need for kidneys and a variety of regional kidney banks have been set up to facilitate in the collection, preservation and rapid distribution of kidneys from donors.

It is estimated that by 1984 some 55,000 persons (in the United States alone) will require chronic hemodialysis. An additional 5,200 patients will receive kidney transplants. All these services combine for a medical cost of some three billion dollars.[1]

The heart transplantation picture is somewhat different. Cardiac transplantation received a considerable notoriety when Dr. Christian Barnard of South Africa made the first human heart transplant in 1967. Since that time a number of centers throughout the world have continued doing heart transplants. Perhaps the most successful of these centers is that at Stanford University Medical Center, under the direction of Dr. N. E. Shumway.

The number of successful heart transplants—success being measured by survival of six months beyond the transplantation event—still is in the few hundreds. However, most heart transplant patients die within a few years. Probably the longest living heart transplant patient has survived about 10 years after the surgery. Apparently, if the patients are carefully selected, they have about a 65% chance of living for one year and 50% chance of living for 5 years beyond the transplantation. In 1978 the cost of the first year of posttransplant care at Stanford University was $50,000. The annual cost of medication and surveillance for subsequent years was about $2,300.[2]

While there has been considerable medical success in the area of organ transplantation, not only with regard to kidneys and hearts but also with other organs and tissues, there are some significant associated moral issues to be considered. At the outset is a fundamental question: Is it morally acceptable to transplant an organ from one living person to another? Another issue relates to the manner in which an organ is obtained from a donor—that is to say, the need of getting a free and informed consent from the prospective donor. A third group of issues has to do with the recipient: primarily, how the recipient is to be selected. This issue became particularly acute regarding heart transplantation, especially in the late 1960s and early 1970s when a fad, so to speak, swept the country. Some hospitals doing heart transplantations had many as 25 recipients waiting for a heart. When a potential heart donor arrived in the emergency room, how was the lucky recipient selected?

---

[1]Guttman, Ronald D., "Renal Transplantation," *New England Journal of Medicine,* Nov. 1, 1979, p. 975.

[2]Schroeder, John S., "Current Status of Cardiac Transplantation," 1978, *Journal of the American Medical Association,* May 11, 1979, pp. 2069–71.

This chapter will briefly consider some medical aspects of organ transplantation, as well as a variety or moral issues associated with this medical procedure.

Some Medical Aspects of Organ Transplantation

The Organs

Among the organs available currently for tissue transplantation are kidney, heart, liver, lung, pancreas, the Islet cells of the pancreas, and skin. Some bone has been transplanted as well as heart-valve leaflets from human or animal sources. *As methods of obtaining and preserving organs improve, there is little doubt that other organs will be involved in transplantation procedures.*

Because an organ is a living system, it needs to be preserved in a viable condition before transplantation. Irreparable damage can readily be done to an organ and to its cells by insufficient oxygen. Transplantation specialists readily admit that there are problems in tissue preservation that they have not yet adequately resolved. While it is relatively simple to maintain in a viable state suspended cells in a deep frozen condition for at least 20 years, this cannot be done for a larger organ.

Keeping cells or tissues at deep-freeze temperatures preserves them because it greatly diminishes their need for oxygen. However, the freezing or thawing process can result in the formation of tiny ice crystals within the cell which will damage or destroy cellular structure. Much of this can be avoided by very rapid freezing and by the use of glycerol, or similar substances, to replace cellular water. However, the larger the amount of tissue, the more difficult it is to get rapid freezing (or thawing) to occur deep within the tissue. For this reason, adult human organs like kidneys or hearts cannot be preserved in a viable state by deep freezing (cryogenic) techniques.

For the present, the best method of preserving the organs involves perfusing them, that is, circulating through the blood vessels of the organs a fluid which is rich in certain electrolytes (intracellular ions) and is kept at a low temperature but above freezing. Human kidneys can be preserved by this procedure for about 72 hours, while hearts can be preserved for approximately 6 hours, and livers for 8 to 10 hours.[3]

---

[3]For a fuller discussion of medical aspects of transplants, see Russel, Paul S. and Cosimi, A. Benedict, "Transplantation," *New England Journal of Medicine*. Aug. 30, 1979, pp. 470–79.

With special equipment it is possible to remove an organ in one city and then to transport it to another city by plane, all the while maintaining its viability by the process indicated above. Thus, with the help of computer-linked informational centers, it is possible to complete successfully more andmore long-distance transplant procedures.

Another concern regarding organ transplantation has to do with what is called histo-compatibility, the ability of one living organism to accept tissues from another. An organ belonging to one individual is a *foreign* organ relative to another, and if introduced into that person's body, it automatically will be rejected. That "rejection system" (the immune response) is part of the same system which fights bacterial infection. Without some way of controlling the rejection, a transplanted organ will not be accepted by the recipient's body; it will cause a severe reaction and require that the organ be removed.

However, there have been developed several drugs which have the property of what is called immunosuppression, that is to say, these drugs suppress the body's immune reaction which would otherwise reject the organ as a foreign invader. These drugs, unfortunately, have the property not only of suppressing the rejection system, but also of interfering with the system responsible for dealing with bacterial infections. While using them, the person becomes vulnerable to infection.

Considerable research is being done in order to find drugs or other substances that will *selectively* suppress the immune system of the body. The goal would be to control rejection of a transplanted organ without interfering with the body's capacity to deal with bacterial invasions. Experiments with animals have given researchers hope that the answers will be found for human beings in the relatively near future.

Another manner of reducing tissue rejection is by obtaining an organ from a person who is genetically close to the recipient. Thus, for example, an organ from an identical twin would not be rejected because both donor and recipient have the same genes. An organ from a closely-related individual, such as a non-twin sibling or parent, is quite likely to be accepted; but it, too, may be rejected in time. By careful tissue-typing, that is to say by matching certain specific characteristics of the recipient's and donor's cells, it is possible to choose an organ which very closely matches the recipient's cellular needs. If there are many individuals waiting for any given organ, one determining requirement would be to find the individual recipient who is most closely matched to the donor organ. This does not necessarily mean that the transplant will be successful, but rather that the use of immunosuppressant drugs may be more effective since they will be used at a lower level.

The Donor

The sources of organs for transplantation are either from cadaver donors (i.e., persons who have just died) or from living donors. An ideal cadaver donor would be one who had been previously healthy, but who suffered death from irreversible damage to the brain. It is best when the donor arrives at the hospital while there is still respiration and heartbeat.

It is also desirable that the kidneys be functioning, that the patient have fixed dilated pupils and no reflexes, not have a history of chronic kidney disease (especially for a kidney donor), and be less than 60 years old. The potential donor also should be free from any systemic disease such as malignant hypertension, diabetes, or generalized hardening of the arteries. The donor should not have any cancer, except perhaps for brain cancer, and should be free of infections. A *most important stipulation is that, in the case of cadaver donors, the diagnosis of death must first be established before any removal of organs be initiated.* (See Chapter 17).

The Recipient

Care must be taken that the recipient has a reasonable chance of surviving the surgery and that suitable tissue compatibility tests have been performed. Furthermore, alternative means of managing the condition should be considered and excluded before entering into the organ transplantation process. Experience has shown that it is advisable to prepare the patient emotionally for the surgery and the post-operative course. Having someone else's organ—especially the heart—in one's body can produce a significant alteration to one's body image.

When there are multiple recipients for a single organ then the choice of the recipient should generally be based on medical reasons over and above all other considerations. The process for making such a choice will be discussed in more detail in the subsequent section.

Moral Issues

Regarding Organ Transplantation Itself

The Catholic Church's basic position regarding organ transplantation can be found in the statements of several popes. Perhaps one of the most recent papal remarks relevant to this issue was made by Pope John Paul I who, in addressing the 7th International Congress of the Organ Transplant Society meeting in Rome, September 1978, greeted them as follows:

> We are content today to express to you our congratulations and our trust, for the immense work that you have put in the service of human life in order to prolong it in better conditions. The whole problem is to act with respect for the person and for one's neighbors, whether it is a question of donors of organs or beneficiaries, and never to transform man into an object of experiment.[4]

Prior to 1978, Pope Pius XII (in 1953 and 1956, for example) had made several statements applicable to this topic. However, in reading the words of Pope Pius XII one should recall that he was writing fresh from the revelations of the medical atrocities that took place in the Nazi concentration camps during World War II. He was concerned that in no way would humans be used again for experimentation or as a convenient "stockroom" for organs.

Pius XII was opposed to one erroneous interpretation of the *Principle of Totality* for justifying morally the removal of organs from one living human being for the benefit of another. This principle itself simply states that *a part of the body which here and now impedes the life or overall well-being of the individual may be removed if there is no other way to provide for the significant benefit for the person losing the body part.* It is a time honored criterion in Catholic moral teaching. But the erroneous interpretation which Pius XII objected to did not require any significant benefit to the *donor.* This interpretation of the principle of Totality, thus, actually opened the door to *Totalitarianism.* This is the all too familiar vision of the individual as having no value except as a useful part of the "total society" or the "total race". The total society or race is personified in some "more important" member to whose needs a "less important" member—or his or her parts— is to be sacrificed. But, the Pope insisted, the human person is not simply a part of society or humanity in the same way as an arm or kidney is part of one physical organism. The God-given destiny of a human person, no matter "how unimportant" in the eyes of others—and the destiny of his or her bodily parts—is not primarily to be disposable for the sake of others.

---

[4]*L'Osservatore Romano,* English Edition, Sept. 14, 1978, p.2.

To defend organ transplant from a living donor to another person, then, Church teaching would require that each and every such donation in *some* way immensely benefits precisely the *donor*, and not only the recipient. Otherwise, the Principle of Totality as Christian tradition has developed it, and indeed, as any soundly-rational humanistic ethic would have it, cannot in truth be invoked.[5]

Pius XII issued his warning against this or any other any totalitarian interpretation of the Principle of Totality in a talk to a group of eye specialists meeting in Rome, May 14, 1956.[6]

While the address focused primarily on transplantation of corneas from cadaver donors, nonetheless, the principles which he describes would be applicable in general to other tissues and organs involved in transplantation. Pope Pius XII takes great care in establishing the appropriate dignity of the human corpse, because it was an abode of the spiritual and immortal soul and also because the dead body is ultimately destined for resurrection to eternal life. He goes on to say:

> On the other hand, it is equally true that medical science and the training of future physicians demands a detailed knowledge of the human body, and that cadavers are needed for this study. What we have just said does not forbid this. A person can pursue this legitimate objective while fully accepting what we have just said.
>
> It also follows from this that a person may will to dispose of his body and destine it to ends that are useful, morally irreproachable and even noble (among them the desire to aid the sick and the suffering). One may make a decision of this nature with respect to his own body with full realization of the reverence which is due to it, and with full attention to the words which the apostles spoke to the Corinthians. This decision should not be condemned, but positively justified.

There has been some division in the past among Catholic theologians about the morality of organ transplantation. But today the major-

---

[5]Marcellino Zalba (*Theologiae Moralis Compendium*, Madrid, 1958, vol. I, n. 1576, ad b, beta): "Many arguments put forth to defend [organ donation] certainly do not prove their point because of: [1] their false comparison [between the individual bodily organism made up of many body parts, and the societal organism made up of many human individuals], or [2] their bad application of the principle of double-effect, or [3] their misuse of the motivation of charity or mystico-moral unity which binds human persons to one another."

[6]Address published in *The Human Body* (Boston, Ma, The Daughters of St. Paul Press, 1960), p. 381.

ity of interpreters understand the words of Pius XII as not truly prohibiting the practice, but as urging restraint, and as insisting that the Principles of Totality not be invoked in an erroneous, totalitarian way. Rather, many moralists argue, a donor's free decision, at least out of charity, to make such a donation does indeed benefit the donor in an immense *spiritual* way, which makes the physical loss *spiritually* worthwhile to the donor, and thus is in harmony with the Principle of Totality.[7] There may even be occasional cases when a mentally-incompetent prospective donor, not capable of the above mentioned truly free decision of charity, would nonetheless benefit from a donation authorized by a proper proxy. For instance, by a proxy's consent, a severely retarded man might give a kidney to save the only living relative he has who regularly visits him. Here, if the *emotional* benefit to the donor justifies the physical privation and perhaps emotional trauma of organ donation, then he is not simply being "used".

Organ donation which in *some* way significantly benefits the *donor* may be made so long as the desired good for the recipient and the reasonably anticipated harm to the donor are proportionate to each other. However, it is equally important that the donor retain a *functional* integrity of his or her body. Thus, the donor may donate one of two healthy kidneys because one fully functioning kidney can provide adequate renal function for the individual under normal circumstances. But, in the name of fraternal charity, the donor cannot freely permit the removal, while living, of his or her heart or of a single kidney if the other one is absent or diseased.

As far as Catholic hospitals, physicians, nurses, or other involved persons are concerned, the issue of organ transplantation is treated, although very briefly, in the *Ethical and Religious Directives for Catholic Health Facilities*, which was approved by the National Conference of Catholic Bishops in November of 1971. Directives #30 and #31 consider the transplantation of organs from living donors and from cadavers.[8] These two Directives read as follows:

---

[7]Zalba (*loc. cit.*) notes: "Perhaps an argument could be made [in defense of organ donation] that the human person does not exceed the limits of a rightful stewardship of his or her own [bodily] substance if, *for his or her own spiritual good*, that person gives to another person the organ this other person needs. For God entrusts to each person [a certain] stewardship over his or her own bodily powers for any action truly useful to that person as a total being. It is not at all clear that [the same God who gives this stewardship over one's own bodily powers] is opposed to the stewardship [of a bodily part] for a *higher* [that is, the *spiritual*] good of the *donor* by a surgery which is not at all necessary to the [*physical* health of the] donor. Such a stewardship seems to be both within the order allowed by God, and indeed in harmony with it." (emphasis added)

[8]Published by the Catholic Health Association, St. Louis, Mo.

130

30. The transplantation of organs from living donors is morally permissible when the anticipated benefit to the recipient is proportionate to the harm done to the donor, provided that the loss of such organ(s) does not deprive the donor of life itself nor of the functional integrity of his body.

31. Post-mortem examinations must not be begun until death is morally certain. Vital organs, that is, organs necessary to sustain life, may not be removed until death has taken place. The determination of the time of death must be made in accordance with responsible and commonly accepted scientific criteria. In accordance with current medical practice, to prevent any conflict of interest, the dying patient's doctor should ordinarily be distinct from the transplant team.

The Ethical Issues Regarding the Donor

As mentioned in the previous medical discussion of organ transplantation, the donor may either be a cadaver or a living donor. In the case of the cadaver donor, it is important that the individual really has died.

Arising from the need of the cadaver donor to be truly dead is the issue of brain death determination. Often the donor would have been maintained on a respirator, and circulation stimulated in order that the organs to be transplanted would be in the best condition possible. A fuller discussion of brain death may be found in Chapter 17. At this point it is sufficient to say that brain-related criteria for the determination of death may be used if scientifically reliable and if properly applied.

Regarding the use of cadavers of anencephalics for organ donation, this procedure would necessarily require brain death criteria which would certify a cadaver. Unfortunately, there is as yet no clear agreement among scientists on such criteria for anencephalics or other neonates. Should the required brain death criteria materialize eventually, then it would seem that, as a general principle, an anencephalic cadaver could be used for organ donation. If tissue or organs are taken from a human fetus while it is still alive, and this normally will cause death, the procedure will fall under the same moral objection as abortion itself.

Even the taking of tissue or organs from *dead* human fetuses generally merits serious moral objection *if these fetuses have been intentionally killed by abortion*. For any organ procurement which intentionally exploits the deliberate killing of an innocent fetal child, also, implies further contempt for that violated life and morally desensitizes and corrupts the society which allows such degradation.

131

The requirement of total brain death for the taking of vital tissues and organs points to serious moral questions regarding one medical procedure which has surfaced in the late 1980's: removal of brain tissue from living fetuses for transplant purposes. Some medical researchers believe, for instance, that such tissue, implanted in the brain of an Alzheimer's or Parkinson's disease victim, brings significant relief. To morally defend such tissue removal, perhaps a solid argument might be possible that the fetal brain could, in some cases, *functionally* be totally dead without all of the individual brain cells necessarily being dead. Scientific data together with careful rational analysis would have to arrive at certainty on this point. Until and unless we have such certainty, however, the inviolability of innocent human life would rule-out such exploitation of a living fetal person. This is obvious, especially, since it would seem that without such reasonable certainty of the fetus' *de facto* death, the brain tissue removal itself clearly would be lethal to the fetus.

In cases of morally-acceptable organ donation it is necessary to have obtained prior release from the donor if a signed statement indicating that the donor is willing to give his organs after death is ideal. On the legal level, the Uniform Anatomical Gift Act, which has passed in all fifty states, does provide for such a pre-death determination to be made. A number of states offer applicants for a driver's license the opportunity to indicate their determination to be organ donors. Such a declaration is then entered on the back of the driver's license. If a donor-release document is not available, then necessary consent must be obtained from the next of kin.

Ethical Issues Regarding the Living Donor

Because the donor has a right to the integrity of his or her body, a properly informed consent must be obtained. In addition, the donor has only limited dominion over his or her body and, consequently, there are certain conditions which must be met before the donor can give an organ. *The donor certainly cannot give an unpaired organ, such as the heart, which will most certainly result in death. This would be equivalent to suicide.*

In addition, the donor does have the responsibility of maintaining the *functional* integrity of his body—if not anatomical. Hence, in the case of paired organs, he may give one kidney providing the other kidney is healthy and able to maintain adequate kidney function for him. Although there has been some loss of anatomical integrity, functional integrity has been retained.

One special difficulty may arise when the prospective donor is a brother, sister, close relative of the recipient, and is reluctant to undergo the procedure. Because of the pressure placed on such a potential donor, it is questionable whether a truly free consent can be given. He or she may know the medical consequences and risks involved in the donation and may be very fearful of going through with it. If the donor individual is married, it may well be that the spouse objects to the donation. Consequently, every effort must be made to make sure that undue pressure is not placed on the potential donor. This requires that the family situation be carefully weighed by those involved in the organ transplantation process before a donor is solicited.

A particular difficulty emerges when the prospective donor is a minor. May the parents volunteer their child's kidney for the benefit of another child's life? *Proxy consent may not be given for the benefit of another individual if there is any more than a truly minimal risk or loss to the donor.*

Moral Issues Regarding the Recipient

Problems associated with the recipient are, in a sense, less acute since it is the recipient who is going to benefit by the process. One decision that needs to be made is whether the intended transplantation procedure truly offers some benefit to the individual. The process of transplantation is not without risk itself and the benefits and risk must be weighed in this situation. The proper informed consent needs to be obtained from the recipient as well.

A relatively sticky problem arises when there are multiple recipients for a single organ. The medical facts must first be determined. Which potential recipient, for example, has the greatest chance of accepting the organ by virtue of tissue compatibility? The issue of recipient selection from a group has been discussed widely. Should social criteria be a factor? Should age, need, or some other fact be involved in the determination of which recipient gets the organ? Would it be proper for a young and otherwise healthy man or woman who has great promise for the future to be preferred over an older individual who is a chronic alcoholic and has relatively little to offer society? Should a mayor of a city, governor of a state, a general, ambassador, or bishop be preferred over someone who is relatively a social nonentity?

Pragmatic reasons cannot be allowed to dominate. As a consequence, some have suggested a lottery method so that the selection among the candidates who are medically and approximately equal would be equitable. There is no simple answer, but it would seem that the basic question would be that of need—who has the greatest need? Even here, there are many factors which are difficult to weigh. Ultimately, the one who has control over the organ disposal is the one who makes the decision.

Conclusion

The beginning of this chapter discussed the fact that there is not intrinsic objection to organ transplantation. Medical progress has been steady in the past 30 years and recent discoveries give promise for the development of even better means of performing successful transplantation procedures. With the aid of an inceasingly well-informed public, the supply of organs from suitable donors is expected to increase. The ethical questions are numerous and complex, but they do not seem to be without solution.

Discussion Questions

1. How would you compare the feasibility of kidney and heart transplants with each other?
2. Why has deep freezing of human organs been impossible up till now?
3. What is the advantage of tissue-typing for successful transplantation of organs?
4. What caused the hesitation of Pope Pius XII to accept transplantations from one living donor to another?
5. What is the moral objection to giving an impaired organ to another as an act of charity?
6. Should a living donor be permitted to select the recipient of his or her kidney when someone else has a greater need and a greater hope of a successful transplant?

Preview of Chapter 12

- Various cultures have approved suicide for the sake of honor or other specific reasons.

- But the world religions of Judaism, Christianity, and Islam have opposed it as destroying God's gift of bodily life.

- If a "right to suicide" were created in the courts, it could easily lead to voluntary euthanasia—killing a person who would request it.

- Just as persons are radically different from animals, mercy killing of persons differs radically from "putting animals to sleep."

- Catholic teaching in the 1980 *Declaration on Euthanasia* hold that the objectionable nature of the act of mercy killing is not changed by the error of judgment of someone who requests it.

- Under American law, euthanasia is a homicide, and both religious and non-religious reasons support that legal position.

CHAPTER 12

Suicide and Euthanasia

The previous chapter explored the increasingly successful transplantation of human organs to preserve the life and health of the recipients. This chapter presents a directly opposite issue. Both suicide and euthanasia take away human life. Yet the possible choice of these practices can be appealing, particularly to persons suffering with terminal illness. These critical moral issues about ending human life must be discussed.

Chapter 5 presented public opinion research which links abortion, euthanasia and suicide. Persons who are willing to accept deliberate killing by abortion to solve personal and social problem also tend to accept euthanasia and suicide to solve personal and social problems. A pro-death ideology has gained strength in recent years in the United States.

What factors might explain this? Perhaps the progress made in providing human comfort has made pain and suffering less tolerable and death more acceptable. Perhaps the success medicine achieves in prolonging the dying process has begun to enhance the attractiveness of a quick death.

Another factor might be an increased emphasis on individual rights which dates back to the civil rights battles of two decades ago. Popular expressions like "the right to die" suggest to some people a civil right to end their life. Seneca, a first century Roman philosopher, described this outlook well:

> Just as I shall select my ship when I am about to go on a voyage, or my house when I propose to take a residence, so I shall choose my death when I am about to depart from life.

However, the constitutional right to life in the United States has not so far been interpreted to assert a right to end one's life or to have a physician end it. Civil rights claims thus far have been limited to the claims of equal treatment before the law. The legal aspects of suicide and euthanasia will be included in the separate discussions here.

Suicide

Suicide may be described simply as an act by which one brings about one's own death. *Experts in ethics of the Catholic tradition usually narrow the description to acts in which death is chosen as a means to an end the person expects to accomplish.* Thus, deaths in mountain climbing or martyrs' deaths do not count as suicide.

Suicide strikes at the common human instinct of self-preservation. It seems clear that the great majority of persons who take their own lives do so because they are so emotionally disturbed that they act compulsively or with greatly restricted freedom of choice. The finality of the successful act of suicide offers no further chance for reflection and deliberation. On the other hand, great numbers of persons who attempt suicide unsuccessfully are actually crying for help, and welcome a new lease on life.

Could the deliberate act of suicide, calmly and reflectively chosen, be judged morally acceptable in certain specific circumstances? Throughout recorded history people of various cultures and world-views have judged that it can. The list includes the ancient Roman Epicureans who justified suicide if life became too painful, and the Stoics who justified it if one might otherwise lose self-control or act in an unworthy fashion. But it also includes all those who accepted the notion that one might need to commit suicide for the sake of honor. Those who have justified suicide have subordinated the instinct of self-preservation to the particular values suicide might achieve.

On the other hand, the world religions of Judaism, Christianity, and Islam have opposed suicide because they regard human life as God's gift which his children are to use as faithful stewards. These religions regard eternal life as a resurrected life with God, not merely the survival of a disembodied soul or an endless reincarnation. Hence one cannot justify suicide as merely a superficial change of condition or an eager leap into eternity. Suicide destroys bodily life and violates stewardship of that bodily life.

Yet some contemporary ethicists who are generally opposed to suicide wish to admit of reasons which may, in some cases, outweigh the evil of self-destruction. Daniel Maguire has adopted such a position.[1] This would mean that suicide could not only be morally excusable because of emotional considerations, but even objectively licit because of the excusing circumstances.

The most common objection to this position rests on its assumption that other values can be actually measured to judge at what point they may outvalue life. A more basic objection rests on its assumption that one may act directly against the basic good of human life. Fathers Benedict Ashley and Kevin O'Rourke have argued that the moral dimension of such acts cannot be set aside.[2] They hold that certain kinds of acts like willful suicide are so opposed to the human person and the order of society that they are irreversibly evil.

Significantly, not all ethicists who are willing to use the method that Daniel Maguire adopts are willing to apply it to cases of suicide and euthanasia. Some of these scholars, as a matter of practical judgment, simply find no good reasons or sufficient values to outweigh the evil of self-destruction.[3]

Catholic teaching on suicide has consistently opposed it without admitting exceptions. For instance, the 1980 *Declaration on Euthanasia* presented a brief synthesis of the teaching:

> *Intentionally causing one's own death, or suicide, is therefore equally as wrong as murder: such an action on the part of a person is to be considered as a rejection of God's sovereignty and loving plan. Furthermore, suicide is also often a refusal of love for self, the denial of the natural instinct to live, a flight from the duties of justice and charity owed to one's neighbor, to various communities or to the whole of society—although, as is generally recognized, at times there*

---

[1]Maguire, Daniel, *Death by Choice* (Garden City, N.Y.: Doubleday, 1974) p. 221.

[2]Ashley, O. P., Benedict and O'Rourke, O. P., Kevin, *Health Care Ethics. A Theological Analysis* (St. Louis, Catholic Health Assoc. 1982, Second Edition) pp. 169–170.

[3]For example, see Ashley and O'Rourke, *op. cit.*, pp. 377–378.

are psychological factors present that can diminish responsibility or even completely remove it.[4]

The psychological factors which diminish *responsibility* for suicide mentioned in the *Declaration* do not refer to excusing reasons which would render the act morally acceptable. They refer to conditions in the subjective order which reduce moral guilt for the evil action. Hence, the pastoral teaching of the Catholic Church has not accepted the theory described above which would sometimes render suicide objectively licit because of excusing circumstances.

Yet this pastoral teaching does suggest genuine concern to assist persons who attempt suicide. In some cases they may have even consciously adopted the theory that excusing reasons exist to justify their suicide. The stewardship of life tradition which prohibits suicide includes a clear responsibility both to care for one's own life and to assist others who are so troubled that they are contemplating suicide.

Obviously this approach would oppose any attempt to create a constitutional "right to suicide." Though states may choose not to make suicide a punishable offense, this does not entail such a "right." The reasons why a state should not encourage suicide have been analyzed in a careful study by Germain Grisez and Joseph Boyle.[5]

If a "right to suicide" were created in the courts, the legalization of *assisting suicide* would follow readily. This would easily, in turn, bring about the legalization of *voluntary euthanasia,* for in voluntary euthanasia a person's desire to have his life ended is honored by a physician or some other person. At present, of course, such acts are prohibited by law.

The public opinion research presented in chapter 5 actually suggested that the American public is more permissive of a physician practicing mercy killing than of individuals committing suicide in the same circumstances. The fact that medical assistance enters into euthanasia cases may make it more socially acceptable than solitary suicide.

Euthanasia

The word "euthanasia" may have a strange ring to it for some people hearing it for the first time or two. From its Greek origins it means

---

[4]Vatican Congregation for the Doctrine of the Faith, June 26, 1980, available from U.S.C. C. Publications, 1312 Massachusetts Ave. N. W., Washington, D.C., 20005, p. 3.

[5]Grisez, Germain and Boyle, Joseph M. Jr., *Life and Death with Liberty and Justice* (Notre Dame, In., University of Notre Dame Press, 1979) pp. 125–127.

"easy death" or "dying well." Taken in that literal sense, the word can have a very positive and acceptable meaning within the stewardship of life tradition.

However, the modern meaning of this word of Greek origins is "mercy killing." Webster's *New Collegiate Dictionary*, Eighth Edition, defines it as "the act or practice of killing individuals that are hopelessly sick or injured, for reasons of mercy." Thus the dictionary definition limits the word to *an easy death because one has been deliberately killed.*

Euthanasia has been standard practice in this active sense of mercy killing for generations—*in the case of suffering animals.* Dogs, cats, cows, racehorses,— all are "put to sleep" when further treatment would be useless or not costworthy. A "mercy hunt" in Florida disposed of 2000 deer who would otherwise have starved.

The fact that humans are not usually "put to sleep" by mercy killing as animals are emphasizes what is already known: Animals and humans are different kinds of creatures. But the mere intuitive awareness of this difference does not immediately explain why human beings do not put one another to death in the face of incurable illness.

What difference does being human make to how one cares for the dying? For one thing, tender, loving care seems not to be found among animals. At least such care is not freely and willingly chosen by animals, or manifested in the intelligent and skillful manner of humans. Human care differs radically from the way animals care for one another.

Moreover, human persons mutually recognize their own common dignity and treasure it, whether sick or well. It seems unlikely that animals can understand their own dignity or their own role in the universe.

In Christian faith, of course, human persons can and do face suffering in union with Christ, instead of choosing death by suicide or euthanasia. But the human capacity for faith arises from the specifically human ability to commit oneself to a belief or a set of values, another aspect of the difference of being human.

In Christian ethics, the practice of mercy killing of a person who requests death raises moral objections comparable to those posed by suicide. If one practices mercy killing on someone without that person's explicit request, an added moral problem arises—that of straightforward murder, even though the murder is committed for an unusual and seemingly high-minded reason.

These ethical objections are linked with the inviolability of innocent life discussed in chapter 4 of this volume. Even when a suffering person requests to be put to death, the act of mercy killing remains a human act directly aimed at destroying the good of an innocent human life. The considerations involved in discussing capital punishment do not apply—the individual has done nothing to forfeit the right to life. *In fact, the suffering person, because of an urgent human need,* has a right to additional care from the human community.

Hence, the unfortunate situation of a person who wishes to be put to death does not change the moral significance of the act of killing, attacking the good of life itself. Human life is not *the supreme* good—God is. But the goodness of human life remains *the basic good of human experience.* Many Christian scholars of ethics have difficulty accepting capital punishment because of this fact. But surely, in the case of suffering persons, the considerations of criminal, anti-social behavior that are cited in capital punishment have no relevance.

As in the case of suicide, some ethicists who are generally opposed to mercy killing wish to admit of reasons which may outweigh the evil of taking innocent life. Their position rests on an analysis of human acts in which acting against the basic good of life can be overlooked because of other values achieved in that action. As mentioned above, their approach presumes some kind of calculus to compute when other values outweigh the good of human life. It also, and this seems to be the core objection, assumes that acts like killing the innocent are not irreversibly evil in themselves. The Catholic tradition holds that such acts are always evil because they are opposed to the human person and the order of society.

The Vatican *Declaration on Euthanasia* of 1980 seemed to address directly this ethical position which could justify euthanasia for proportionate reasons:

> It may happen that, by reason of prolonged and barely tolerable pain, for deeply personal or other reasons, people may be led to believe that they can legitimately ask for death or obtain it for others. Although in these cases the guilt of the individual may be reduced or completely absent, nevertheless, the error of judgment into which the conscience falls, perhaps in good faith, does not change the nature of this act of killing, which will always be in itself something to be rejected.[6]

The reference to the fact that an error of judgment does not *change the nature of this act of killing* teaches very plainly that euthanasia cannot be justified for proportionate reasons. Authors like William May who have entered the proportionalism debate have said that, "Although we are not obliged to ward off death at all costs, we are obliged to love life

---

[6]*Op. cit..* p. 5.

and should not deliberately and of set purpose regard life as evil or as a non-good."[7]

Acts of mercy killing carry the same significance as acts of suicide—they violate reverential stewardship of the gift of human life. Mercy killing does violence to the person killed, it does much more than merely provide a superficial change from earthly life to life after death. Some who find reasons to justify mercy killing think of it as "merciful release" from bodily existence. But this view actually devalues bodily life and misrepresents the human condition in which body and soul reciprocally interact and influence each other.

Catholic teaching on euthanasia was not newly discovered in time for the 1980 *Declaration* mentioned above. The United States bishops had minced no words in their 1976 pastoral letter on the moral life. "It is a grave moral evil deliberately to kill persons who are terminally ill or deeply impaired," they wrote. "Such killing is incompatible with respect for human dignity and reverence for the sacredness of life."[8] And, of course, the Second Vatican Council included euthanasia in its list of crimes against the person along with "willful suicide".[9]

The public opinion research viewed above in chapter 5 showed general public approval of doctor-administered voluntary euthanasia rising from 36% in 1947 to 59% in 1977, a span of just 30 years. This could well coincide with the dimming of the public's memory of Nazi involuntary "euthanasia" in the period before and during World War II in Germany.

Dr. Leo Alexander, a consultant at the Nuremburg trials after World War II, wrote a revealing analysis of "Medical Science Under Dictatorship," describing how at least 275,000 persons were euthanasia victims.[10] The victims were persons who were mentally or physically handicapped, including children. The classification for euthanasia was broadened to include children who were bed wetters or designated "difficult to educate."[11]

Obviously, a state-administered euthanasia program such as this represents a terrible abuse of the principle of voluntary euthanasia. Yet the core principle of all euthanasia remains the same: Killing is a remedy for suffering or for a useless existence. The moral opposition to all

---

[7]May, William E., *Human Existence, Medicine, and Ethics*, (Chicago: Franciscan Herald Press, 1977) p. 133.

[8]*To Live in Christ Jesus*, (Washington, D. C.: U.S.C.C. Publications, 1976) p. 20.

[9]*The Church in the Modern World (Gaudium et Spes)*. #27.

[10]*New England Journal of Medicine* 241: 39–47, 1949.

[11]Wertham M. D., Fredric, *A Sign for Cain*, (N.Y., N.Y.: Warner Paperback Books, 1966), p. 175.

euthanasia, voluntary, involuntary, and nonvoluntary (killing those unable to be consulted) utterly rejects that core principle.

Pope Pius XII rejected it in 1943 in his encyclical letter *Mystici Corporis* (The Mystical Body).[12] The heroic German Protestant theologian, Dietrich Bonhoeffer, rejected it too. Bonhoeffer, who was himself executed by the Nazis, argued that if one is truly concerned about a suffering person, one will not kill that person without consent. And, furthermore, a suffering person may not give such consent without incurring the guilt of suicide, which is at bottom a sin of lack of faith. Bonhoeffer cites as a Biblical foundation for his rejection of euthanasia the *Exodus* text, "The innocent and the just you shall not put to death." (Ex. 23:7)[13]

This strong moral rejection of euthanasia obviously relies heavily on religious belief which considers God as the Lord of life and all created persons as stewards, holding their own lives and the lives of others in sacred trust. Some persons who find no transcendent meaning or plan in the universe feel that suicide is no more absurd than the world itself. Other profound thinkers like Albert Camus have struggled with absurdity, but concluded that, "Even if one does not believe in God, suicide is not legitimate."[14] *Without relying on traditional religious faith, the famous concentration camp doctor, Viktor Frankl. reached the conviction that, "The so-called life not worth living does not exist".*[15]

Faced with differing opinions on the ethical justification of euthanasia, and with especially strong sympathy for voluntary euthanasia in the face of terminal illness, what is and what should be the position of the law?

Euthanasia and the Law

Under American law euthanasia is a homicide. Even though the person who performs the act of mercy killing bears no ill will toward the person killed, if the one who kills can comprehend that his conduct is prohibited, the necessary malice for homicide is present. It is true that juries have often treated with great leniency persons who perform mercy killing, sometimes accepting the defense of temporary insanity.

---

[12]New York, Paulist Press Edition, # 104.

[13]Bonhoeffer, Dietrich, *Ethics*, (N. Y.: Macmillan, 1965) pp. 160–66.

[14]Camus, Albert, *The Myth of Sisyphus* (Transl. by J. O'Brien, N.Y.: Vintage Books, 1955) p. v.

[15]Frankl, Viktor, *Psychotherapy and Existentialism* (N.Y.: Washington Square Press, 1967) p. 129.

Legislation to legalize voluntary euthanasia under some form of judicial control with a duly appointed euthanasia referee was proposed in England in 1936. Similar statutes have been proposed elsewhere and no doubt will continue to be suggested in the years ahead.

In the legal battles over abortion, the proponents of liberalized abortion laws often argue that people who have religious or moral obligations need not practice abortion. The proponents simply wish to give legal support to "freedom of choice." However, the fact that an unconsenting and unborn human being is killed offers strong opposition to this "freedom of choice."

Predictably, the "freedom of choice" argument will be heard even more forcefully in favor of voluntary euthanasia. Should not the law sustain a suffering person's freedom of choice to have his or her life ended? People who have religious or moral opposition to euthanasia need not exercise that choice.

Strong arguments against legalizing voluntary euthanasia which argue from non-religious premises can be presented. Such statutes would permit private individuals to take the lives of other private citizens—a massive compromise of society's commitment to protecting human life. The impact on the medical profession would be enormous—killing would become an alternative to medical care. Sick and elderly people would be plagued with the prospect that their time for mercy killing may have arrived. Persons who realize that they have become a burden to others would feel increasingly pressured to choose death. The opportunities for abuse by manipulating a person's consent, especially to the benefit of heirs, would be plentiful.

A more basic objection to legalized euthanasia underlies the practical considerations just listed. If euthanasia should become a public function of society, the liberty of citizens who abhor it to avoid responsibility for such killing will be infringed. Grisez and Boyle offer a thorough discussion of this and other objections to legalized euthanasia in their solid and scholarly study, *Life and Death with Liberty and Justice.*[16]

Because of the "pro-death ideology" referred to in chapter 5 above, the issue of legalizing euthanasia will continue to attract media and public attention. In a previous publication of the Pope John Center, lawyer Dennis Horan cited the major organizations lobbying for the so-called "right to die."[17] Much sympathy for legalizing euthanasia arises from fear of unbearable suffering in terminal illness. Lord Ragland, who introduced a British euthanasia bill in 1969, said later that he would not have introduced it if

---

[16]*Op. cit..* especially chapters 6 and 8.

[17]*The New Technologies of Birth and Death* (St. Louis, MO.: The Pope John Center, 1980, distributed by Franciscan Herald Press, Chicago) pp. 150–153.

he had been aware of what hospices can do in relieving the suffering of terminal illness.[18]

Conclusion

Do many people who contemplate suicide or mercy killing today really want to be killed? One doctor's wise comment was that he met many patients who felt they would be better off dead, but none who wanted him to kill them. The *Vatican Declaration* described the pleas of gravely ill people for death as, "almost always a case of an anguished plea for help and love."[19] The real need, it added, is for love, the human and supernatural warmth with which the sick person can and ought to be surrounded.

Such loving care need not prolong a person's dying by medical treatments which offer no reasonable hope of benefit. The next chapter will explore prolonging life decisions. But in closing this discussion it must be noted that omissions of reasonable medical treatment with the intention of causing death are both ethically and legally equivalent to killing. Thus the category of mercy killing must include killing by intentional neglect. Responsible stewardship of human life both prohibits killing innocent persons and obliges to loving care for them.

Discussion Questions

1. How would you explain the appearance of a pro-death ideology in the United States and in the world in recent years?
2. Can you suggest some non-religious reasons to oppose suicide?
3. If reasons of relieving suffering do not change the nature of the act of mercy killing, how can capital punishment be justified?
4. Why would Albert Camus and Victor Frankl oppose euthanasia?
5. Can you suggest some non-religious reasons why voluntary euthanasia should not be legalized?
6. Can one practice mercy killing by omission of medical treatment?

---

[18]Lamerton, Richard, *Care of the Dying* (London: Priory Press Ltd., 1973) p. 96.
[19]*Op. cit.*. p. 5.

Preview of Chapter 13

- Some forms of medical treatment are more extensive than a norm of reasonable care of human life would dictate. Foregoing such treatment should not be considered ending life.

- The Catholic tradition describes these forms of treatment as ethically extraordinary.

- Two criteria to identify such medicines, treatments, or operations are: the excess burden they might cause and the lack of reasonable hope of benefit.

- If a treatment itself is successful and beneficial, it does not become extraordinary simply because the patient is handicapped or experiences a low "quality of life."

- Persons acting as proxy for those who are not competent to make decisions must always choose ethically ordinary treatments.

- Proxy representatives may forego ethically extraordinary treatment if that would be the patient's wish, or where sound medical judgment indicates that competent patients would also forego the treatment.

CHAPTER 13

Decisions About Prolonging Life

The previous chapter might well have been titled, "Decisions About Ending Life." A human life can be deliberately ended by omission of care or nourishment as well as by acts of direct killing. If a human life is intentionally ended by omission of reasonable human or medical care, such a decision can indeed be judged equivalent to acts of direct killing. Such forms of omission were included in the previous chapter.

However, this chapter will discuss omissions of medical treatment from a new perspective. What if some forms of medical treatment are omitted because, in given circumstances, they are more extensive than a norm of reasonable care would dictate? We are leaving behind the "intention" to end life, whether by act or omission. We now focus on the fact that some medical means used to prolong life may be ethically optional. A decision to forego such means for that reason should not be considered a decision to end life.

Thus even though a person does not wish to end life, he or she still needs to make prolonging life decisions. Generally, people experience an instinctive desire to live. On this basis they tend to request whatever medical treatment will prolong their lives.

On the other hand, the proverbial saying, "The cure is worse than the disease," indicates that people have probably always hesitated to choose some forms of medical treatment. The wonderfully expanding 20th century practice of medicine, of course, has opened great new vistas of possible medical treatment. It has heightened interest in the subject of this chapter.

Furthermore, the effort to decide whether a given medical treatment, such as chemotherapy for a malignant cancer, is "reasonable" immediately poses a question. The question: "Reasonable in whose judgment?" Obviously, the basic answer should be: "Reasonable in the judgment of the sick person."

But sick persons realize that truly reasonable judgments cannot be made in a vacuum. Individuals need some appreciation of the common sense judgment of others in deciding what is reasonable.

Spontaneously, many patients depend on their physicians to help them decide. They ask, "Doctor, what would you decide if you were in my situation?" Doctors are blessed with the most complete information about the medical outcomes of proposed treatments, and they should be the first persons consulted.

But then, how do doctors decide? The intense medical training they receive does not itself equip them to do this. For decisions to prolong life often involve human value judgments which, in turn, presume some coherent framework for making such judgments. They are made consistently only with the help of such a framework.

Furthermore, the stewardship of human life ethical tradition used in this volume teaches that *responsible stewardship of human life obliges people to the use of the "reasonable" means of prolonging life.* It only admits of a genuinely arbitrary decision about other procedures.

Hence this chapter will look for a coherent frame of reference in deciding what are "reasonable" means of prolonging life. It will avoid two extremes. In the one extreme, people simply avoid the medical profession altogether (not a very common extreme in developed countries today). In the other extreme, people judge that all possible medical treatment is "reasonable" and even morally obligatory (this extreme seems attractive to those who value human life, but it actually ignores the norm of "reasonableness" and is becoming increasingly unrealistic).

Our discussion will begin with the Catholic tradition on the reasonableness of medical treatments and then explore the two basic criteria it proposes. This will include some simple cases and the special challenge of improper use of "quality of life" considerations. Finally, the chapter will raise the most crucial difficulty in these decisions, the role of a proxy to represent noncompetent persons for whom prolonging life decisions must be made.

The Catholic Tradition

The Catholic tradition on prolonging life decisions can be found in an ethical directive for Catholic health facilities:

> 28. Euthanasia ("mercy killing") in all its forms is forbidden. The failure to supply the ordinary means of preserving life is equivalent to euthanasia. However, neither the physician nor the patient is obliged to the use of extraordinary means.[1]

Note that this ethical directive has provided a set of terms to identify what are morally obligatory means of prolonging life: "ordinary" means of preserving life, compared to "extraordinary" means. The 1980 *Declaration on Euthanasia* of the Sacred Congregation for the Doctrine of the Faith referred to this classical distinction.

The Vatican statement agreed that as a principle this distinction still holds good. But it frankly admitted that the distinction is less clear today, *"by reason of the imprecision of the term and the rapid progress made in the treatment of sickness."*[2]

Historically, Catholic ethical scholars have been discussing the extent of one's moral obligation to preserve life and health since at least the Middle Ages. A 16th century Dominican, Francisco De Vitoria, exemplifies the attempts to describe what is the extent of reasonable care.[3]

Vitoria speaks of the moral obligation to make whatever efforts people "regularly" make to care for life and health. One would not be obliged, he writes, to invest one's life's savings in medicine nor to buy the most expensive foods, even if they were the healthiest. He summarized his teaching, saying, "One is not held to employ *all the means* to conserve his life, but it is sufficient to employ the means which are of themselves intended for this purpose and appropriate."

---

[1] *Ethical and Religious Directives for Catholic Health Facilities,* approved by National Conference of Catholic Bishops, Nov. 1971. Printed by Catholic Health Association of U.S., St. Louis, MO 63134.

[2] *Declaration on Euthanasia,* Vatican Congregation for the Doctrine of the Faith, June 26, 1980. (Washington, D.C., U.S.C.C. Publications) p. 8.

[3] For a historical study of this principle, see *Moral Responsibility in Prolonging Life Decisions* edited by Donald G. McCarthy and Albert S. Moraczewski, O.P. (St. Louis, MO, Pope John Center, 1981, distributed by Franciscan Herald Press, Chicago), chapter 7.

The first scholar to discuss surgery for prolonging life, another 16th century Dominican named Domingo Soto, talked about amputation of an arm or leg. Anesthesia was not available in those days, and Soto said firmly that no one was morally bound to endure such torture to prolong life.

The ethical reflection that developed within the Catholic tradition took account of individual and subjective considerations in deciding what was ordinary care. Several authors noted that a person who experienced intense dislike of a certain food need not eat it, although it would otherwise serve as an obligatory means of preserving life. Likewise a woman who experienced intense embarrassment being examined by a male physician need not submit to the examination.

Yet, these authors did not reverse their judgment when individual circumstances made certain procedures more feasible. Thus no moral obligation bound wealthy people to use more expensive medical treatment than what was reasonable for ordinary people.

Hence the ethical tradition which accompanies the notion of ordinary and extraordinary means of prolonging life relies on a common sense judgment to determine what is reasonable or ordinary. Exceptional circumstances may excuse from the general norm but they do not, in other cases, make it even more binding.

The United States Catholic Bishops summarized this ethical tradition in contemporary language in 1976:

> While euthanasia or direct killing is gravely wrong, it does not follow that there is an obligation to prolong the life of a dying person by extraordinary means. At times the effort to do so is of no help to the dying and may even be contrary to the compassion due them. People have a right to refuse treatment which offers no reasonable hope of recovery and imposes excessive burdens on them and perhaps their families. At times it may even be morally imperative to discontinue particular medical treatments in order to give the dying the personal care and attention they really need as life ebbs. Since life is a gift of God we treat it with awesome respect. Since death is part and parcel of human life, indeed the gateway to eternal life and the return to the Father, it, too, we treat with awesome respect.[4]

---

[4]*To Live in Christ Jesus,* A Pastoral Reflection on the Moral Life, National Conference of Catholic Bishops, Nov. 11, 1976. (Washington, D.C., U.S.C.C. Publications Office, 1976).

Two Criteria

Two phrases in the bishops' statement identify two basic criteria for distinguishing extraordinary from ordinary means of prolonging life. The two phrases are *"no reasonable hope of recovery"* and *"excessive burdens."*

The latter consideration, excessive burden, claimed much attention in the ethical speculation of the Catholic theologians described above. In fact, Father John Connery in the Pope John Center research study, *Moral Responsibility in Prolonging Life Decisions,* points out that the primary determination of ordinary or extraordinary means rested on that question.[5] The general norm for excessive burden is the common reaction of ordinary people, even though some individuals' feelings may make their burdens heavier in specific cases.

Theologians included *great expense* as an index to "excessive burden," even though health cannot really be measured in terms of money. They simply meant that common sense could judge when an expenditure became excessive for an individual or family. Today, the public and private reimbursement systems have overshadowed this consideration.

Nonetheless, an individual may still find treatment costs excessive and hence "extraordinary." Furthermore, it may become increasingly imperative to find some way of limiting the tremendous sums now being reimbursed for extensive health care treatment in specific individual instances. This, of course, will pose grave concerns of justice and fairness.

Two other comments about the "burden" of health care treatment are significant. First, the burden may *vary greatly* when a procedure like hemodialysis is used for a brief period as opposed to an indefinite period. Secondly, a procedure may be *medically routine* and ordinary and still impose an *excessive burden* on the patient, as when hemodialysis becomes a treatment of indefinite duration for a person in declining health.

By this reasoning, tube feeding and hydration sometimes could be judged morally extraordinary and therefore non-obligatory. A competent patient would have a right, therefore, to refuse a long term imposition of this technological substitute for natural ingestion. Also, provided that removal of such tubal support does not cause significant discomfort or other burden, this judgement would apply to patients medically identified as, beyond reasonable doubt, irreversibly comatose.

Some Catholic physicians and moralists, accept this view. Others challenge it. They consider supplying food and fluids as simply basic care, regardless of how modern technology may have to deliver these to

---

[5]*Op. cit.*, chapter 9, especially pp. 127–134.

the patients. Up to the writing of this revised edition, the Church has made no statements except to encourage further discussion of this issue.

The other phrase used in the U.S. Bishop's statement to identify an extraordinary means of prolonging life was "no reasonable hope of recovery." Father Connery, in the essay mentioned above, discusses this concern under the heading of a "useless" means of prolonging life. Past theologians were speaking primarily of the uselessness of prolonging terminal illness. This means that a mere prolonging of the dying process can be considered extraordinary.

Father Gerald Kelly S.J. became a leading Catholic expert on these questions in the pre-Vatican II period of modern medical ethics. He covered the category of a "useless" means of prolonging life by speaking of a means which "would not offer a reasonable hope of benefit." Hence his definition of an extraordinary means is this:

> Extraordinary means are all medicines, treatments, and operations, which cannot be obtained or used without excessive expense, pain, or other inconvenience, or which, if used, would not offer a reasonable hope of benefit.[6]

An obvious example of Fr. Kelly's means "without reasonable hope of benefit" would be a rather limited hope of successful surgery. Thus, only a 40% chance of successful back surgery or a 40% chance of a successful kidney transplant would seem to qualify these procedures as ethically extraordinary, because of such limited hope of benefit. *Medically, these procedures may be quite routine and common.*

The whole spectrum of medical treatments for serious heart conditions and various forms of cancer offers multiple examples of treatments with a doubtful "reasonable hope of benefit." The spectrum will include a goodly number of treatment situations where sincere and conscientious people will differ on the existence of a reasonable hope of benefit. Here persons faced with decisions should take wise counsel, but realize the latitude which exists. From the perspective of one's moral obligation before God to preserve life it would seem that, generally speaking, a doubtful obligation does not bind in conscience. Patients may, of course, still choose treatments without feeling bound to do so.

However, the criterion of "without reasonable hope of benefit" can be used in an improper way. *Note that, if a medical treatment successfully accomplishes its purpose, this normally constitutes reasonable hope of benefit.* It

---

[6]Gerald Kelly, S.J., *Medico-Moral Problems* (St. Louis, MO, The Catholic Hospital Association, 1957) p. 129.

may be the case that, even after successful treatment, a patient does not enjoy normal health or a normal "quality of life." This unfortunate situation should not be the basis for considering the treatment ethically extraordinary.

For example, a blind person may have appendicitis. The fact that the appendectomy will not restore eyesight gives no reason for considering it ethically extraordinary. On the contrary, an appendectomy today usually offers great hope of benefit and would usually be considered ethically ordinary.

Thus, as a matter of principle, the distinction of ordinary and extraordinary means of prolonging life should not be used in a discriminating way against handicapped people. If a medical treatment does not correct one's diminished quality of life, the treatment does not thereby become ethically extraordinary. However, Father Connery pointed out, in the essay already mentioned, that *if the medical treatment itself diminishes one's quality of life, this will often give reason to consider it ethically extraordinary.*

For example, a person who would experience greatly reduced mental alertness because of surgery for a brain tumor might well consider the surgery ethically extraordinary. It could be considered excessively burdensome without reasonable hope of benefit. However, a woman of low I.Q. should not consider removal of a breast tumor ethically extraordinary when the surgery has a high prospect of success. The treatment offers a reasonable hope of benefit, it does what it is designed to do, even if it will not raise her I.Q.

Although the criterion of "without reasonable hope of benefit" may be used improperly in cases like this last one, the criterion itself remains helpful. It applies particularly to cases of persons in the final stages of terminal illness. Here, indeed, the "benefit" may be nonexistent if the person is dying a painful death.

The Vatican Declaration on Euthanasia discussed this very situation:

> When inevitable death is imminent in spite of the means used, it is permitted in conscience to take the decision to refuse forms of treatment that would only secure a precarious and burdensome prolongation of life, so long as the normal care due to the sick person in similar cases is not interrupted.[7]

These reflections on "Two Criteria" for judging whether a medical treatment should be considered ethically extraordinary reflect particu-

---

[7]*Op. cit.*, p. 10.

larly the long and developed Catholic tradition on this matter. However, a much wider consensus can be found in both the ethical and medical communities, despite variations of terminology.[8] But this issue becomes especially difficult when a proxy must represent noncompetent persons in prolonging life decisions.

The Role of Proxy Consent

This chapter began by asking what kind of treatment to prolong life the norm of "reasonable" care would dictate. It made clear that competent patients must participate in the decisions about their treatment, even though they should be guided by the common sense judgments of others. They may, of course, choose more aggressive treatment than the common sense standard would propose. But they should hesitate to choose less aggressive treatment, if they accept the moral obligation to take reasonable care of their lives.

What about infants, or patients who have become incompetent to decide for themselves, or adults who have always been mentally incompetent?

Clearly, in the stewardship of life tradition, *the parent, relative, or guardian who acts as proxy has a responsibility to provide ethically ordinary means of prolonging life*. To choose otherwise would violate the Christian command to love one's neighbor and the underlying principle of justice to the neighbor. The act of injustice automatically violates charity.

A parent who would not consent to an appendectomy for a child, whether because the child were retarded or simply unwanted, would seem to deny an ethically ordinary medical treatment. Similarly, a husband or wife who would refuse emergency surgery which could save the life of their unconscious spouse would seem to violate the same norm of justice and charity.

This anchor principle cannot solve all difficult cases. Consider some other possibilities. The person giving proxy consent may know that the patient wishes to forego ethically extraordinary procedures and that the noncompetent patient considers the possible treatment extraordinary. Unless the person acting as proxy is convinced that the treatment is really an ordinary one, that person could surely be morally justified in

---

[8]For example, Paul Ramsey, *Patient as Person* (New Haven, CT, Yale University Press, 1970) and *Dying*, Considerations concerning the passage from life to death, Task Force on Human Life, Anglican Church of Canada, edited by Lawrence Whytehed and Paul Chedwick (Toronto, Can., The Anglican Book Centre, 1980).

refusing the possible treatment for the patient. This point is clearly illustrated in the Brother Fox case (see chapter 15), although Fr. Eichner had to go to court to get legal approval for following Brother Fox's wishes.

Perhaps the *patient's actual wishes* about ethically extraordinary treatments are not known or cannot be known, and whether the patient would *judge a treatment ethically extraordinary* is also unknown.

The two unknowns here can be treated separately, taking the second first.

1) *Is the treatment ethically extraordinary?* Surely some cases can be known to be ethically extraordinary without the patient's own judgment. The more obvious of such cases would be, for example, prolonging a painful death by using a respirator or increasing suffering by a traumatic procedure like amputation, if it offered no appreciable benefit or significant prolongation of life. In such cases the judgment that a procedure is ethically extraordinary rests heavily on a purely medical evaluation of the procedure. The person acting as proxy could be guided by sound medical judgment in such cases.

2) Still, even in the cases just mentioned, the other unknown remains. *Would this patient perhaps choose extraordinary treatment?* Under the supposition that nothing is known of the patient's own disposition, ethicists tend to consider "the best interests" of the person, which can be judged from what competent persons would decide in comparable or parallel situations.[9]

This last unknown, the patient's own disposition, raises the question of Living Wills. Such documents are statements people may sign which say that in circumstances with no reasonable expectation of recovering from extreme mental or physical disability they do not wish to have their lives prolonged by medications, artificial means, or heroic measures. One ethical concern with this language comes from the fact that artificial means can even include artificial nourishment. This introduces a very difficult and sensitive question both legally and ethically. However, if the document merely records a person's general disposition and is not subject to legal binding force, this question of terminology has no great consequence.

On the other hand, legislating a legal binding force for these documents raises grave questions, discussed in chapter 15 of this volume. Furthermore, in the judgment of many ethicists and lawyers, such legislation is unnecessary, unwise, and would leave people without signed Living Wills in an awkward position.

---

[9]See Connery, *op. cit.*, pp. 131–132.

Signed statements without legal binding force can still assist proxy representatives by clearing up the second unknown just described. The Catholic Hospital Association of the United States in 1974 published a "Christian Affirmation of Life" to assist people in recording their disposition to forego ethically extraordinary means of prolonging life. A new, briefer version of this document was published in 1982 by the Catholic Health Association with the sub-title, "A Statement on Terminal Illness."[10]

Conclusion

This chapter attempted to present a coherent framework for making prolonging life decisions in a reasonable way and in accord with respect for human life. Admittedly, such decisions are sometimes unclear and disputable. Two practical guidelines may help:

> 1) Competent patients must judge whether a procedure is extraordinary as they would make any conscious decision, with consultation, reflection, and prayer. Even though they judge a treatment to be at least probably extraordinary, they may still conscientiously decide to undergo it.
> 2) Proxy representatives of incompetent or noncompetent patients must not hesitate to provide ethically ordinary treatment. Furthermore, they may only forego extraordinary treatment according to the disposition of the patient or, lacking that information, where sound medical judgment indicates that competent persons would also forego the treatment.

The next chapter will consider some "hard cases" of prolonging life decisions. Meanwhile, let it be said in conclusion, as Paul Ramsey has said so well, that

> Together, medical men and moralists need most urgently to renew the search for a way to express both moral recoil from any arbitrary shortening of life, and moral recoil from any arbitrary prolongation of dying.[11]

---

[10]Available from Publications Dept., Catholic Health Association of the U.S., 4455 Woodson Rd., St. Louis, MO 63134; 10¢ each.

[11]Ramsey, *op. cit.* p. 156.

Discussion Questions

1. Why should not all medical treatment be morally obligatory in the stewardship of life tradition?
2. Is omitting ethically ordinary treatment equivalent to killing?
3. Can you suggest some concrete examples of excessive burden in medical treatment?
4. Why should expense be included as an indication of burden?
5. What are examples of treatment that does not offer reasonable hope of benefit?
6. In what sense are parents "free" to decide what medical treatment should be provided for their children?

Preview of Chapter 14

- Case studies are essential in applying the theoretical principles about ethically extraordinary means of prolonging life. Eight cases are briefly presented.

- Hildegarde F. had two amputations because of diabetes at the age of 79. These procedures could readily be considered ethically extraordinary because of the burden for a person of her age and health.

- Mrs. B., a 70 year old woman with deteriorating health, decided to forego hemodialysis, the mechanical substitute for kidney function. This decision can be justified as foregoing an ethically extraordinary treatment.

- Dr. R. was kept on a respirator even after he became comatose with terminal cancer. The attending physician may have had good reasons for this, but it was not ethically obligatory.

- Wilhelm K. was seriously ill in an Intensive Care Unit. His family requested no heroic measures but the staff disagreed and persuaded the family not to give up. The staff felt Wilhelm wanted their treatment, even if it was heroic.

CHAPTER 14

Hard Cases of Prolonging Life Decisions

Introduction

A television series entitled "Hard Choices" recently dramatized difficult issues in medical ethics. Admittedly, hard choices exist, but only because of hard cases—actual situations where moral values or moral norms seem to conflict. The previous chapter presented a largely theoretical view of an ethical framework for making prolonging life decisions. This chapter will explore some practical cases, most of which are fictionalized versions of real situations, in the light of that theory.

The importance of case studies on prolonging life decisions emerges readily by recalling the two criteria discussed in the previous chapter, "excess burden" and "without reasonable hope of benefit." Only by looking at real situations can one estimate what those modifying words "excess" and "reasonable" mean in the common sense estimate of normal people.

Those who would make these estimates within the stewardship of human life tradition of Catholic teaching and the Judeo-Christian heritage particularly need what one theologian called, "purity of heart." What he meant was a reverence for the uniqueness and transcendence of human life which rules out mercy killing and intentional ending of life by omission. In this disposition one recognizes that sickness and suffering are both inescapable and redeemable in the human condition. Hence one does not focus first on suffering and then how to escape it. Instead one should ask which medical options are morally acceptable and at the same time minimize suffering.

In responding to each of the cases below, relevant questions will be raised, often indicating that the case should have been presented more fully. But the brief cases still make key points. At the end, two legal cases will be introduced from an ethical perspective but they will reappear in the next chapter on "The Law and Withdrawing Treatment."

The first series of cases will concern competent patients, the second noncompetent patients.

Competent Patients

Hildegarde F.

Hildegarde F. came to the nursing home at the age of 78. Her husband of the same age was still living, but could no longer care for her. She had four children who all remained in touch with their parents and were living in the area. Her husband remained in the family home but spoke of coming one day also to live at the nursing home.

Her main physical problem was severe diabetes. The summer after she came to the nursing home, she was hospitalized with a serious ulcer on her left leg and a bypass graft was performed. By that fall she was showing obvious signs of physical weakening, becoming non-responsive and almost comatose. Then, through an unusual set of circumstances, she got a different physician. He studied her problems and the non-healing ulcers on her right leg with abscesses and early stages of gangrene. He recommended amputation.

The family and Hildegarde decided in favor of the amputation. It was performed that winter and she came through the surgery beautifully. She returned to her alert and cheerful personality. In fact, she was getting around so nimbly that the following fall she broke her hip. She was bedfast as a result.

The following summer her left leg began showing the same conditions as the right had earlier. The same doctor who had recommended the earlier amputation again recommended amputation. The family showed less reluctance than the last time, probably because of her previous great recovery. However, she died in the hospital after the amputation.

Is amputation of a leg an ethically extraordinary procedure? It surely was in the 16th and 17th centuries, when performed without anesthesia and antibiotics. Today it can obviously be done much more efficiently, even for a 79 year old woman with severe diabetes.

However, our estimate of an excessive burden would incline to include the first and, even more definitely, the second amputation for Hildegarde. Therefore, she could have decided against these procedures without an unreasonable neglect of the gift of life.

The fact that she chose both procedures manifests that even procedures that go beyond the ordinary can be successful, helpful, and rewarding. Hildegarde derived great benefit from the first amputation.

Foregoing ethically extraordinary treatment can often shorten life, as foregoing the first amputation surely would have.

In Christian faith, many people of Hildegarde's age don't mind this. They are lonely and look forward to a different life with God and their loved ones who have died. But Hildegarde could still enjoy the visits of her husband and four children. She apparently felt that heaven could wait! Fortunately, she could herself participate in the decisions about amputation. Possibly, if she could not have, her family would still have made the same choices, knowing her will to live.

Mrs. B.

Mrs. B., a 70 year old woman with deteriorating health, had been receiving hemodialysis, the mechanical substitute for kidney function. The procedure was particularly difficult for her since her blood clotted easily and there were difficulties in the maintenance of the necessary shunt. She indicated her desire to forego hemodialysis. In their concern for a truly informed consent, her physicians set up an interview at a time when her system would be most free of poison which might cloud her judgment. After a frank and open discussion, they accepted her decision to cease hemodialysis.

This brief case does not convey the pathos that must have surrounded Mrs. B.'s decision. In contrast to the previous case, no mention is made of her family. Nothing is said of her financial capabilities, although in the United States special federal funding has supported hemodialysis since 1974. The brief reference to "deteriorating health" tells very little of her actual physical and emotional condition.

161

However, the case makes clear that she considered the prospect of continual dependence on hemodialysis an excessive burden. Medically, it was extra difficult for her. As in the amputations above, we incline to agree with a judgment of excessive burden. However, even more obviously than in the case of foregoing the amputations, foregoing hemodialysis will shorten Mrs. B.'s life. Could her decision even be considered suicidal?

The doctors worried about the decision she was making. Perhaps they even raised the question of suicide with her. Presumably, she did not consider her decision suicidal.

Inasmuch as a person simply intends to forego an excessive burden caused by prolonging life treatment, that person has no suicidal intention. The death which occurs results from the diseased kidney rather than any lethal acts. Hence, presuming that Mrs. B. had no suicidal intention, the chief ethical concern rests with her judgment of the excessive burden. Presuming again that she could only expect continual dialysis, with its attendant difficulties, for the rest of her life, she did not decide unreasonably.

Calvin P.

Calvin P. is only 52 years old, but has suffered from multiple sclerosis for 15 years and had to retire from his job as a machinist two years ago. He had become morose and withdrawn. He attempted suicide by slashing his left wrist and was admitted to the hospital. He was cooperative and alert in the Intensive Care Unit but insisted he wanted no supportive treatment. A consulting psychiatrist discovered that his mother-in-law had recently received a diagnosis of inoperable cancer. The psychiatrist helped him and the family deal with the grave emotional issues. Calvin had subconsciously resented the loss of attention to his own problems. He soon retracted his request for no supportive treatment.

This brief case does not present Calvin's full medical condition or the prognosis of his multiple sclerosis. It simply makes clear that his initial disposition to forego supportive treatment came from his depression. Hence the case was handled very helpfully within that context.

Calvin's condition of multiple sclerosis has handicapped him and forced his retirement. However, the medical treatment for his attempted suicide and the routine care he receives for his condition do not automatically become ethically extraordinary.

When and if some specific treatment for Calvin became a significant burden, the ethical criteria discussed in chapter 13 would become relevant. Meanwhile, Calvin's situation manifests the importance of family relationships in patients' decision-making. It shows that the ethical principles about prolonging life decisions may easily be misapplied in the face of emotional crises.

Lucy H.

Lucy H. was 56 years old and had received outpatient chemotherapy for cancer of the lymph nodes affecting her central nervous system. She came to the hospital because of a seizure and cardiac arrest. An Intensive Care Unit staff review with the family resulted in continued aggressive care. This was based on her previous excellent response to chemotherapy, and Lucy's often stated desire to survive until the birth of her first grandchild.

Many of the ICU staff felt that continued therapy was not warranted and "inhumane." A smaller group of ICU staff, plus her daughter and Lucy herself, wanted to continue as long as there was hope. Many hours of staff meetings were devoted to the decision to stop or continue. Lucy slowly survived complications and was discharged after seven weeks. At home she was able to engage in daily activities around her home without limitations. She saw the birth of her granddaughter, enjoyed Christmas and New Year's, but died suddenly 11 weeks after discharge.

The last 18 weeks of Lucy's life are described in this case. She spent 7 in hospital treatment and the last 11 weeks at home, enjoying the Christmas holidays and becoming a grandmother for the first time. The case portrays the attitude of many staff persons in ICU who obviously knew her hopeless condition and saw good reason to consider aggressive treatment ethically extraordinary.

The ethical framework for prolonging life decisions presented above would tend to support their judgment. Both the hopelessness of her condition and the burden of further aggressive treatment could be cited. One would readily focus instead on pain relief and relieving a patient's anxieties in a case like Lucy's.

But, even if ethicists would find grounds for not considering aggressive treatment obligatory, Lucy still wished it. She had her own reasons which her pregnant daughter supported.

As the case turns out, the seven weeks of treatment provided Lucy with a considerable benefit. Perhaps if the staff who opposed aggressive treatment could have foreseen that, those many hours of staff meetings could have been shortened. Lucy's treatment seems to have been ethically extraordinary but humanly very rewarding.

Noncompetent Patients

Dr. R.

Dr. R. had practiced in St. Z. Hospital for 30 years and was now a patient there, dying of cancer. He had been put on a respirator by his friend, the attending physician. After he became comatose his wife and his son, a practicing lawyer, requested that the respirator be removed. The physician refused, even after the administrator of the hospital seconded the request. Dr. R. survived another week and then expired while still on the respirator.

A clear consensus seems to have developed in both the ethical and legal community that respirator treatment need not be used to prolong the lives of patients in the final stage of terminal illness. Hence, an immediate response to this case might be great disappointment at the stubbornness of Dr. R.'s friend and attending physician.

Unfortunately, background information which might explain his conduct is missing. For instance, could Dr. R. have exacted a promise from the attending physician never to "give up" on him? Since the case mentions no such promise, it may be that the attending physician simply couldn't decide to take a step that might be considered "abandoning" a colleague.

Realistically, the attending physician may have been more concerned about legal repercussions, even after the hospital administrator gave reassurance. However, the likelihood of legal charges or liability in Dr. R.'s case seems extremely slight. Medical policy has become increasingly clear. The House of Delegates of the American Medical Association in 1973 adopted this statement: "The cessation of the employment of extraordinary means to prolong the life of the body when there is irrefutable evidence that biological death is imminent is the decision of the patient and/or his immediate family."[1]

The next chapter will discuss thoroughly the legal aspects of withdrawing a treatment such as a respirator. Fortunately, the legal consensus seems to have accepted the ethical judgment that withdrawing a useless treatment should not be considered killing, even though death occurs. In Dr. R.'s case it seems clear that the respirator was a useless treatment. Of course, if he *had* insisted on its use, his choice should have been respected.

---

[1] *Journal of the American Medical Association* 227 (1974) p. 728.

Mrs. T.

Mrs. T. was a 72 year old woman living in a nursing home. When the physician discovered a small but malignant tumor on her breast he recommended immediate removal and felt sure he could remove it completely. Mrs. T.'s daughter persuaded her to refuse the surgery, possibly because of her own fear of hospitals. Mrs. T. died a rather painful death after seven months.

Mrs. T.'s case does not belong with noncompetent patients except that she apparently allowed her daughter to decide against the surgery for her. Since the cancer of Mrs. T.'s breast led to a rather painful death, it must be assumed that the surgery would have prevented some of her suffering, even if not totally successful. On this grounds of benefit and possible cure for the patient, the surgery could easily be judged an ethically ordinary treatment.

The patient's rights seem to have been violated by her daughter, as the case is described. Surely the daughter's fear of surgery or hospitals was irrelevant. Had the mother felt this same fear, of course, it could have made the surgery extraordinary for her. This would be an individual and subjective consideration like the ones mentioned above in the preceding chapter.

Mildred D.

Mildred D. came to the nursing home at the age of 77, a widow with two sons who visited her faithfully at least every week. During 18 years in the nursing home, Mildred seemed content and lived rather serenely. Her physical condition held up fairly well but her medical records showed arteriosclerotic heart disease, secondary anemia, a history of an abdominal mass of undetermined origin and atrophy of her larynx and esophagus, secondary to stroke.

After her 94th birthday, she experienced increased difficulty in eating and swallowing, and became more and more frail. The doctor directed a soft diet because of her problem. She herself remained calm and indicated she was ready to die and go to the Lord. In fact, she refused more and more to make the effort to eat, and became so debilitated that she was confined to her bed.

Her eating problems got worse instead of better. Finally the doctor told her sons he wanted to try a nasogastric tube to give her some nourishment. She resisted this almost from the beginning. Despite her disorientation, she knew what it was, and simply didn't want it. She pulled it out numerous times and each time the re-insertion was more painful for her. Her doctor suggested restraints to keep her from pulling it out. Somehow in the space of three weeks she managed to pull it out at least 15–20 times.

The staff at the nursing home knew Mildred well—after 18 years she was almost a charter resident. They felt it was cruel to keep inserting the tube she didn't want. A conference was held with her sons, the physician, and a pastoral care advisor. It was agreed that something should be done. A solution was reached: the tube would not be removed, but the restraints would be. The next time Mildred removed the tube, it would stay removed. That whole day she was left unrestrained and she left the tube in. But that evening she removed it and it stayed out.

The staff continued offering what nourishment they could, primarily ice cream, for 7–10 days. The doctor was uncomfortable about her increasing malnutrition. He suggested that a gastrostomy tube could be inserted in her side at the hospital under local anesthetic if the sons wished. They hesitated several days but their mother was still lingering and they decided to authorize the tube. It was inserted but it didn't work too well. The staff did their best to provide the most comfort possible to Mildred. She died three weeks after the tube was inserted, aged 95 years and 8 weeks.

This case graphically pictures the particularly agonizing dilemmas sometimes faced because of artificial feeding. An instinctive outlook shared by many people views nourishment as the most ordinary of human needs. When modern technology can meet that need for helpless people, must it not always respond promptly and effectively?

The ethical analysis presented in this volume leaves room for some exceptions to such a response. The clearest example of an exception might be the situation of prolonging the dying process of a comatose cancer victim with intravenous nourishment. Many responsible ethicists in the stewardship of life tradition would insist only on relieving possible dehydration with a liquid IV containing very little nourishment.

In support of this logic one can argue that the death of such a patient results from cancer rather than intentional neglect. The parallel argument could be made that Mildred died because of the atrophy of her larynx and esophagus, not from intentional neglect.

Those responsible for Mildred's care obviously did not want to cause her death. The decision not to remove the nasogastric tube but simply wait for her to do so indicates this. The doctor's final suggestion about inserting the gastrostomy tube in her side does too.

While Mildred's condition differed greatly from that of a cancer victim, it was also hopeless in a medical sense. In the basic ethical tradition used here, it seems the tube need not have been inserted in Mildred's side as long as she could be kept comfortable and avoid dehydration.

166

On the other hand, the genuine concern to avoid seeming neglect or deliberate starvation is important. The general public has not yet drawn clear lines to distinguish when failure to supply nourishment artificially is ethically acceptable and when it constitutes neglect. The courts will be called upon also to deal more fully with this issue. The legal precedent established thus far and described in the next chapter simply has not authorized foregoing of food and drink.

Wilhelm K.

Wilhelm K., a 76 year old man, had surgery for an abdominal condition. While in the Intensive Care Unit he told the staff of his eagerness to return to his vigorous and active life. Before experiencing the stomach problem, he had been in good general health.

However, he developed a stomach infection, blood poisoning, and pneumonia. He required a tube for breathing and became delirious from the blood poisoning. His family requested that no heroic measures be undertaken.

The ICU staff, however, felt his condition was reversible. When they set up a meeting to review the case, the family refused to attend. Subsequently, the family reluctantly agreed to aggressive efforts with a daily re-evaluation. Wilhelm was unresponsive to their efforts and died on the 18th day of his hospitalization.

This case shows the dynamics of family-staff relationships. Apparently the family gave up hope before the professional ICU staff did. Families today may well be influenced to this by the widespread modern attention to prolonging life situations and the popular slogan of "death with dignity."

From the limited medical information presented here one might judge that the medical staff acted rightly. Even if one were to argue that their efforts were ethically extraordinary, they were relying on Wilhelm's own desire to get well. While the family were surely closer to him than the ICU staff, the family may have been following their own intuitions, rather than Wilhelm's own wishes.

This case might serve as an example of a common oversimplification of the ethically appropriate approach to these decisions. The family may have been correct in judging the aggressive treatment ethically extraordinary, but a second consideration remains. Namely, if the treatment is extraordinary, what evidence exists of Wilhelm's disposition to forego it? Some evidence exists that he wished it.

Only when no evidence exists to indicate whether or not a patient wishes ethically extraordinary procedures should the proxy representa-

167

tive fall back on considering the patient's best interests or what competent people would consider the best interests. Wilhelm's case did not conform fully to that model.

Infant Doe and John Storar

Both these cases are discussed in the following chapter on the law and withdrawing treatment. It would be best to turn now to pages 188–190 and read these cases. John Storar was an adult who had never been mentally competent and Infant Doe did not live to reach the use of reason. Both cases, then, involve proxy decisions about life-prolonging measures which were reached without participation of the patient.

Good reasons can be given why the medical procedures should have been considered ethically ordinary in both cases. Infant Doe could have survived with corrective surgery. This was refused and he was not even given intravenous nourishment long enough for a thorough judicial review of the case.

Very possibly the controlling reason why Infant Doe was denied surgery came from his retarded condition. He was a victim of Down's Syndrome, but it could not yet be known whether he belonged to the small fraction of such children who are severely retarded. His case seems to exemplify the improper use of quality of life considerations described in the previous chapter. As corrective surgery, his treatment had a strong hope of benefit. It would not have cured Down's Syndrome, but that should not have been a factor.

John Storar's case involved blood transfusions which would compensate for blood loss due to internal bleeding. He was terminally ill with leukemia, but apparently not in the final stage of his illness. Thus an ethicist would have difficulty arguing that the transfusions were prolonging a dying agony. The final court decision in New York ruled that John Storar's mother, acting as his proxy, could not refuse the transfusions.

In neither of these cases could the courts argue from the actual dispositions of the patient to refuse treatment. The only consideration could be the treatment itself. Nor could either patient add subjective considerations to influence the judgment that the treatments, in his case, were ethically extraordinary.

It seems the courts would be well-advised to protect the rights of patients to treatment in these cases. Ethically, there are strong reasons to consider the treatments ordinary because of benefit to the patient. The next chapter will explore the legal status of this entire question.

Discussion Questions

1. Have you personally known a case similar to one of the cases in this chapter?
2. Would it have made any difference if Mrs. B. did not begin having hemodialysis treatment?
3. Could a subjective state of mental depression make a medical treatment ethically extraordinary for someone like Calvin P.?
4. Is it possible that Lucy's treatment was more successful than the staff anticipated because of her will to live?
5. Would you have reacted differently than Mildred's sons when they decided to authorize a gastrostomy tube?
6. Do you think the staff were correct in feeling that Wilhelm K. would wish heroic or aggressive efforts to save his life?

Preview of Chapter 15

- Two basic legal doctrines in this chapter are the patient's right to refuse treatment and the use of "substituted judgment" for the noncompetent patient.

- Various state courts have authorized withdrawing or withholding various kinds of medical treatment in various circumstances.

- Infant Doe in Bloomington, Indiana, was denied treatment which would have saved his life in a decision heavily criticized as denying his rights.

- In the Brother Fox case the patient had indicated a disposition to forego ethically extraordinary treatment and the courts supported this.

- In the John Storar case the adult patient had never been competent. The final appeal in New York supported his right to blood transfusions, despite his cancer.

- Living Will legislation may be carefully drafted, as in California, or poorly drafted, as in Arkansas.

CHAPTER 15

The Law and Withdrawing Treatment

In the United States today courts and legislatures are searching for an appropriate scheme of laws and legal principles to govern the termination of medical treatment. Physicians must have sufficient freedom to practice their profession. Families must be free to assume responsibility for the care of incompetent members and children. Yet, if the law is to protect the rights and interests of all citizens, it must not countenance mercy killing or failure to supply reasonable medical care to the sick and handicapped.

In recent years judges and legislatures have moved toward a consensus on applying key legal principles to the termination of medical treatment. This chapter will review these principles and discuss their application in two New York cases. It will briefly survey the living will legislative movement and end by summarizing the emerging legal consensus.

Basic Legal Principles

The two basic legal doctrines underlying termination of treatment are the right to refuse treatment and the use of a "substituted judgment" in behalf of a noncompetent patient.

Under common law, the right to refuse treatment reflects the autonomy of persons in society. In *Satz v. Perlmutter,*[1] the Florida Supreme Court in 1980 held that a 73-year-old patient, mortally ill from amyotrophic lateral sclerosis (Lou Gehrig's disease), could knowingly direct his removal from a respirator, even though it was certain that death would follow in an hour. The court found that a patient has a right to refuse life-preserving treatment especially when it is extraordinary and the patient suffers a terminal illness. Courts, however, have qualified the right to refuse treatment in some instances. Protecting the interests of children who would be orphaned if their parents were not given emergency, life-saving treatment is a case in point.[2]

In the famous case of Karen Quinlan in 1976, the New Jersey Supreme Court went beyond the common law right to refuse treatment by citing a *constitutional* right of privacy as including the right to refuse extraordinary medical care.[3] It held that this constitutional right must be balanced against the state's traditional interest in preserving life. The court decreed that Karen's father, as guardian, could consent to removing her respirator since she was assumed to be terminally ill and the state's interest in preserving her life had diminished because of Karen's chronic vegetative and comatose condition.

The New Jersey Supreme Court did not clarify exactly why it was necessary to develop a *constitutional* right to refuse treatment in the light of the already well-established common law right. The constitutional doctrine seems to have been adopted in the hope of better solving the special problems in cases where persons cannot communicate their consent to or refusal of treatment. Dennis Horan recently pointed out serious objections to making the right to refuse treatment a constitutional right.[4]

In the case of patients who are incompetent due to a chronic comatose condition or mental disability, courts have employed "substituted judgment" in behalf of these persons. For example, in the case of Jo-

---

[1]*Satz v. Perlmutter,* 379 S. 2d 359 (Florida, 1980).

[2]Application of President and Directors of Georgtown College, 331 F. 2d 1000 (1964).

[3]In Re Quinlan, 70 N.J. 10, 40, 355 A. 2d 647, 663–664, *cert. denied sub. nom. Garger v. N.J.,* 429 U.S. 922 (1976).

[4]Horan, Dennis J., J.D., "Euthanasia, the Right to Life and Termination of Medical Treatment: Legal Issues," *Moral Responsibility in Prolonging Life Decisions* (St. Louis, MO, Pope John Center, 1981), pp. 168–173.

seph Saikewicz in Massachusetts the courts in 1977 held that the judgment of a court-appointed guardian could be substituted for that of the 67-year-old man with an I.Q. of 10.[5] The guardian is to consider the best interests of the patient and, as nearly as possible, make the same decision the incompetent patient would have made if he or she had been able to decide upon a course of treatment.

In Massachusetts, the *Saikewicz* decision stated that court approval must be sought in substituted judgment decisions. The *Quinlan* court in New Jersey had said the judgment could be approved by a hospital "ethics committee." Subsequently, a Massachusetts court stated that physicians will not automatically be liable for a lawsuit if they withdraw treatment without judicial approval, nor will they be automatically immune from such liability if they obtain court approval.[6] But in what circumstances do the courts approve a substituted judgment to withdraw treatment?

Circumstances Justifying Withdrawal of Treatment

Courts have generally held that treatment may be withdrawn from incompetent patients only in a severe condition of terminal illness. Thus, in the *Saikewicz* case the Massachusetts Supreme Court limited withdrawal of treatment to those cases where the patient: 1) has an incurable and terminal illness, 2) where there exists no life-saving or life-prolonging treatment, or 3) where such treatment, if available, would only effect a brief and uncertain delay in the natural death process.

Thus, in a subsequent Massachusetts decision in 1980 the state supreme court considered the case of Earle Spring, a 77-year-old man suffering from end-stage kidney disease and chronic organic brain syndrome (senility).[7] The court repeatedly characterized Mr. Spring's disease as incurably fatal and permitted withdrawal of hemodialysis treatment as merely life-prolonging and not life-saving. The treatment offered no prospect of a cure or even a recovery of competence.

A physician's order, "Do not resuscitate" (DNR), effectively withdraws one form of emergency medical treatment. Under such an order health care professionals will not employ mechanical means of resuscitation if a patient suffers cardiac or respiratory arrest.

---

[5]*Superintendent of Belchertown State School v. Saikewicz*, 373 Mass. 728, 370, N.E. 2d 417 (1977).

[6]405 N.E. 2d at 120–122.

[7]Matter of Spring, 405 N.E. 2d 115 (Mass., 1980).

A Massachusetts appellate court in 1978 found a DNR order appropriate in the case of Shirley Dinnerstein, a 67-year-old woman with Alzheimer's disease, who had also suffered a stroke and was in an essentially vegetative state, immobile and speechless. The opinion of the court emphasized that the patient's prognosis was hopeless and that death must soon come.[8]

In a more recent case, a Massachusetts appellate court upheld a similar DNR order in the case of an infant born with severe handicaps.[9] However, in a 1981 case in Minnesota a DNR order was rescinded in the case of Sharon Siebert, a middle-aged woman who suffered severe complications during brain surgery, resulting in brain damage and near-total paralysis. Jane Hoyt, a friend of Mrs. Siebert's, challenged the order, since she was not terminally ill, and a Minnesota State District Court agreed.[10]

One court decision, that of the Delaware Supreme Court in *Severns v. Wilmington Medical Center* in 1980, included a long series of questions which seem to indicate that the judges wondered whether termination of treatment amounted to the legalization of mercy killing.[11] *And, indeed, if termination of treatment of incompetent persons who are not terminally ill is allowed for "quality of life" reasons, the door is open to legalized mercy killing.*

Just such a case made headlines in April, 1982.[12] Physicians diagnosed Infant Doe, born in Bloomington Hospital (Indiana) as afflicted with Down's Syndrome with additional abnormalities of the esophagus that required corrective surgery. The parents refused to consent to surgery and were supported by their obstetrician and the hospital. The infant was also deprived of food and water (the abnormalities made digestion impossible) or even intravenous nourishment and hydration, and died at the age of six days.

A circuit court judge in Monroe County, Indiana, pronounced that the decisions to withhold surgery and nourishment were a proper exercise of parental authority and medical judgment. The Monroe County prosecutor brought action under the child abuse statues and private parties sought to adopt the child and order the life-saving surgery. An appeal was taken to the Indiana Supreme Court, but turned down in a 3–1 decision.

In fact, Infant Doe was not dying and there existed a frequently performed surgical procedure which would have been beneficial. Withholding surgery

---

[8]*Ibid.*
[9]In Re Custody of a Minor, _____ N.E. 2d _____ (Mass. App. Ct., 1982).
[10]*Hoyt v. St. Mary's Rehabilitation Center* (Dist. Ct., Hennepin County, Minn., Opinion date, February 13, 1981).
[11]421. A. 2d and 1334 (Del., 1980).
[12]*NRL News,* May 10, 1982.

and, especially, all forms of nourishment, is not supported by the principles of the *Quinlan* and *Saikewicz* cases. This was not a terminal case until the decision to withhold surgery and nourishment made it one.

Other courts have made the proper distinctions and ordered beneficial treatment for infants in dangerous situations. In the *Baby Houle* case in 1974, a Maine Court was faced with a situation similar to that of Infant Doe. It appointed a guardian to give consent for the corrective surgery against the wishes of the parents.[13] In 1979 in the *Cicero* case, a New York court ordered corrective surgery for an infant born with spina bifida.[14]

Finally, in the famous *Chad Green* case in 1978, the Supreme Court of Massachusetts affirmed a lower court decision to take custody of this 20-month old child away from his parents who refused to consent to chemotherapy for his leukemia.[15]

These three cases illustrate legal precedents for the providing of treatment to incompetent infants which is both life-prolonging and life-saving. *The legitimate State's interest in protecting the lives of all its citizens takes precedence over the parents' right to withdraw or refuse treatment for their children.* A careful examination of two New York cases questioning withdrawal of treatment will help clarify the legal principles under discussion.

Two New York Cases: Brother Fox and John Storar

Brother Joseph Charles Fox, S.M., an 83-year-old member of the Society of Mary, suffered a massive cardiopulmonary arrest during a routine operation in October, 1979. He suffered profound, irreversible brain damage, remained in a coma for four months, and then died, despite the continued assistance of a respirator.[16]

Brother Fox's religious superior, Father Philip Eichner, S.M., requested the hospital and attending physician to remove the respirator. When his request was denied, he petitioned a county court to be appointed guardian of Brother Fox with power to direct the withdrawal of the respirator. At the hearing Father Eichner cited prior statements by Brother Fox that he did not wish extraordinary means to sustain his life should he fall into an irreversibly comatose condition like that of Karen Quinlan.

---

[13]*Maine Medical Center v. Houle*, No. 74–145 (Superior Court, Cumberland, Maine, decided February 14, 1974).

[14]In Re Application of Cicero, 421, N.Y.S. 2d 965 (S. Ct. 1979).

[15]Custody of a Minor, 375 Mass. 733, 379 N.E. 2d 1053 (Mass., 1978).

[16]In Re Eicher (Fox), 102 Misc. 2d 184, 186, 423 N.Y.S. 2d 580, 584–587.

The trial court ruled that Brother Fox's statements were an exercise of the common law right of self-determination and should be honored. The court concluded from the medical evidence that the respirator could only extend the process of dying and the interests of preservation of life would not be compromised by the respirator's withdrawal. This court found it unnecessary and unwise to base its decision on the constitutional right of privacy.

This decision was affirmed by the Appellate Division of the Nassau County Supreme Court.[17] *But they wrote a very different type of opinion,* relying on the *Quinlan* doctrine of a constitutional right of privacy. The court ruled that the right to die in dignity is protected by the right of privacy and that, even if Brother Fox had not expressed his own preference as he had, the substituted judgment of a court-appointed guardian could have exercised the constitutional right to die in his behalf.

The court's opinion went further than any earlier decision in defining a "right to die." In the step-by-step type of development that is characteristic of the law, this small step from a right to refuse treatment to a "right to die" opens the way for courts to fashion a constitutional right to die. *This could well bring about the legalization of mercy killing.* Giving the power to exercise the right to die to parents and guardians of incompetent persons under the principle of substituted judgment offers enormous potential for abuse.

Recognizing such potential abuse, the Appellate Division required that any decision to withhold life-preserving treatment must be sanctioned in a court of law. It also limited the application of substituted judgment to cases where the patient is terminally ill with only an extremely remote probability of ever regaining cognitive brain function. It decided that Brother Fox's case met these criteria. The district attorney then appealed the case to New York's highest court, the Court of Appeals.

The Court of Appeals linked the Brother Fox case with the case of John Storar, a 56-year-old adult with a mental age of two years. Storar had been institutionalized all his life in a state hospital in Rochester and now suffered with terminal cancer. His mother, his court-appointed guardian, at first consented to frequent blood transfusions to compensate for blood loss due to internal bleeding, and then asked for them to be stopped.

The hospital petitioned the Monroe County court for authority to continue the transfusions. The county court followed the recent opinion of the Appellate Division in the Brother Fox case and decided that John Storar had a constitutional right to refuse further blood transfusions,

---

[17]*Eichner v. Dillon,* 73 A.D. 2d 431, 461, 472, 426 N.Y.S. 2d 517, 540, 548 (1980).

which right his mother could exercise on his behalf. The Appellate Division upheld this decision and it came to the highest state court, the Court of Appeals.

The Court of Appeals resolved both cases without employing the constitutional right to privacy that the lower courts had used, following Massachusetts and New Jersey.[18] It supported the Brother Fox decision on the common law right of self-determination which the original county court had used.

On the other hand, the Court of Appeals rejected as "unrealistic" any attempt to decide whether John Storar, if he were competent, would want the potentially life-prolonging transfusions discontinued. His mother could consent to his medical treatment but not deprive him of it. The decision asserted the State's interests in protecting the health and welfare of the incompetent patient.

The decision said in part that the blood transfusions were like food—they would not cure the cancer but they could eliminate the risk of death from another treatable cause. The decision spelled out a principle of great significance. "A Court should not in the circumstances of this case allow an incompetent patient to bleed to death because someone, even someone as close as a parent or sibling, feels that this is best for one with an incurable disease."

This New York Court of Appeals decision may become a model for addressing such cases in the future. *It demonstrates that principles of the common law can resolve difficult medico-legal cases rather cleanly without introducing the complexity inherent in applying constitutional law doctrines.*

This decision also pointed out that neither common law nor existing statutes require judicial approval of decisions to withdraw treatment. This safeguard had been made mandatory in the constitutional law approach of the lower appellate courts. The decision simply offered an optional procedure whereby those in charge of incompetent patients may apply to the courts for a ruling on the propriety of conduct which might seriously affect their charges.

The decision stated that any mandatory procedure for various approvals of decisions to discontinue treatment, including court approval, should come from the legislature. So far, however, legislative action has primarily concerned living wills.

In the last five years, some court decisions have seemed to favor the legal acceptance of euthanasia. For example, a 1985 New Jersey Supreme Court case concerned 84-year-old Claire Conroy who, though only minimally conscious and responsive, was not comatose or in a vegetative state. The decision would have allowed her nephew to have tube

---

[18]438 N.Y.S. 2d at 275, 420 N.E. 2d at 73.

feeding and hydration removed (she died from other causes before this could be carried out). But along with points which we have defended above, the court unfortunately declared also that the handicapped condition of Claire Conroy's life could indicate that her life was not worth supporting.[19]

In another case, A California higher court not only defended the right of Elizabeth Bouvia to refuse, as significantly burdensome, the prospect of long-term tubal feeding and hydration, but also included justices' opinions open to or actually advocating a right to suicide and euthanasia.[20] While publicly defending a patient's right to refuse long-term subjection to man-made contrivances for delivering food and fluids, Los Angeles' Archbishop Roger Mahoney protested the euthanasia-oriented reasoning of the court.[21]

One must keep in mind that, not only the concluding decisions of judges, but also the reasoning behind these enter into our system of law as being, in various degrees, authoritative. Thus the California decision very likely will be cited by some lawyers and judges in the future to legitimate suicide and euthanasia. In contrast, however, California citizens in May, 1988, refused to support a referendum favoring suicide.

Living Will Legislation

Since the California Natural Death Act of 1976, many states have passed legislation empowering a person to write a legally binding directive for the purpose of withholding medical treatment should the person become incompetent.

The more carefully drafted versions of such statutes provide that nothing in the statute is to be construed to condone mercy killing or a deliberate act or omission to end life other than to permit the natural process of dying. But even such statutes fail to consider a physician's own medical judgment if they set up a mandatory duty to withdraw treatment. *Furthermore, the great majority of patients are unlikely to ever exe-*

---

[19]Supreme Court Case of New Jersey, no A-108, September term, 1983 . . . in the matter of Claire C. Conroy . . . decided January 17, 1985.

[20]In the Court of Appeal of the State of California, Second Appellate District, Division Two. 2nd. Civ. No. BO19134, Elizabeth Bouvia, petitioner, v. Superior Court of the State of California for the County of Los Angeles, respondent.

[21]"Two Statements on the Bouvia Case" [a short, preliminary one, and a second, more extended one, both by Archbishop Roger Mahoney of Los Angeles] in *The Linacre Quarterly*, February, 1988, pp. 83–88.

cute a "living will" and physicians may be reluctant to withdraw or with-hold life-sustaining treatment without an official directive.

The California statute tries to bypass this latter problem by provid-ing that the bill does not cancel any previously-existing right to effect the withdrawal of life-preserving medical treatment. However, the Ar-kansas statute, on the other hand, simply states that "all laws or parts of laws in conflict with this Act are hereby repealed!"[22]

The Arkansas Act shows the dangers of such poorly drafted legisla-tion. It does not define terms like "artificial, extreme, or radical method." It does not limit withdrawal of treatment to terminal illness. It allows a parent or guardian to execute such a directive refusing treat-ment for anyone, even a minor, who is mentally incapable of executing one or is "otherwise incapacitated." The Act opens the door to unimag-inable abuse.

To avoid passing legislation which denies incompetent persons their right to life and equal protection of the law and which implicitly autho-rizes mercy killing, certain safeguards are necessary. Such legislation must prohibit mercy killing and assisted suicide, it must be effective only in truly terminal cases, it must not permit withdrawal of basic nourishment or ordinary medical means which are beneficial, and con-sent forms must be truly voluntary. These safeguards are in accord with an emerging legal consensus on termination of treatment decisions.

Since 1983, there has been a growing movement to abandon living will legislation in favor of a legal arrangement much more open to abuse; a wide ranging and binding "durable power of attorney". This power would be given in advance through a patient's directive and would authorize a proxy to have life support removed, with the view of termi-nating the patient's life, should the patient later become incompetent. The decision of the proxy would have full legal recognition.

An Emerging Legal Consensus

The judicial activity recorded in this chapter, bewildering as it may seem on first reading, shows an emerging consensus on legal principles to be applied in termination of treatment situations. Two helpful points of legal consensus emerge:

1) *For the incompetent patient medical treatment may be terminated by a physician when the treatment offers no medically reasonable hope of benefit.* In that situation, treatment such as mechanical respiratory assistance may

---

[22]Ark. State. Ann. Sec 82–3801–3804 (1977).

be terminated and the patient allowed to die as the natural consequence of the underlying disease process.

This means that physicians are not obliged to render continued therapy which does not and cannot improve the prognosis for recovery. Even if the therapy is necessary to maintain the stability of the patient's condition, it should not be mandatory where the ultimate prognosis is hopeless. On the other hand, legal precedent does not permit discontinuing ordinary means of life-support, such as food and drink, because the ultimate prognosis is hopeless.

2) *Likewise, the physician who withdraws treatment from the terminally ill patient for whom death is imminent should not be held criminally or civilly liable for such conduct.* This means that the "treatment" merely unduly prolongs the dying process and its withdrawal merely allows the underlying disease or illness to run its inevitable course.

Note, however, that these two points of consensus apply to a limited class of cases. The "treatment" to be withdrawn is a regimen of medical care, not food and drink. *Furthermore, the cases must be genuinely "hopeless" and the treatment "useless" in the sense that nothing more can be done for the patient and the only sensible course is to withdraw treatment.*

In cases where a physician's judgment rejects treatment which is both truly life-saving and therapeutic, there is no immunity from legal intervention. Thus, this consensus does *not* approve withholding treatment from a handicapped infant who requires emergency surgery because of a life-threatening condition. Such a decision is not based on the inevitable death of the infant but on a judgment that the unfavorable prospective "quality of life" of the infant justifies the omission.

Fortunately, the court in the *Saikewicz* case specifically rejected "quality of life" considerations from playing any part in the decisions by others to withdraw treatment from a minor incompetent person. Thus, any omission based on "quality of life" grounds (which constitutes a genuine form of mercy killing), whether in the case of handicapped infants or senile senior citizens, was condemned in American law.

The *Dinnerstein* case confirmed the principle that in the ordinary and usual case where a patient is dying the choice of treatment is the physician's—there is no need for court authority to make medical judgments. The law remains prepared to deal with an abuse of medical judgment by neglect or mercy killing.

The two New York cases decided jointly by the Court of Appeals each confirm a principle. The *Brother Fox* case clarifies the competent adult's common law right of self-determination to refuse medical treatment, without recourse to the Constitution and complex judicial interventions. The *John Storar* case shows that self-determination does not extend automatically to the parent or guardian of an incompetent patient, and does not allow them to withhold beneficial medical treatment.

As noted above, since 1985, several court decisions have held also that a less than normal "quality of life", in itself, can be reason for abandoning life support. In the Bouvia case, the court favored even a right to suicide and active euthanasia in such cases. Thus, the judiciary's former protection of handicapped persons seems to be eroding somewhat. In contrast, during the same period, one New York State Court of Appeals decision—Mary O'Connor—rejected diminished "quality of life" as justifying withdrawal of artificial life support.[23] Also, in California, attempts failed to initiate a referendum to gain popular approval for suicide in such cases and euthanasian attempts to assist it.

Conclusion

The courts and legislatures exercise their proper function when they set our society's standards for obligatory medical treatment, as discussed here. The two principal points of consensus pointed out here permit withdrawal of medical treatment in either of these cases:

—Where medical treatment will only uselessly prolong the dying state without hope of recovery or benefit, or

—When death is imminent and there exists no life-saving medical intervention.

Finally, a court proceeding should only be required where there is a dispute whether these standards have been violated. These standards should be applied equally to all patients, infants and aged, handicapped and non-handicapped. *While in some respects these legal standards are less flexible than the ethical criteria of chapter 13, they will prevent the legalization of mercy killing and protect every innocent human person's dignity and inviolability.*

Discussion Questions

1. Should the law permit legally competent patients to forego ethically ordinary means of prolonging life?
2. Should the law permit proxy representatives to rely only on oral statements made to them by patients when they were competent?

---

[23]October 14, 1988

181

3. What is the objection to treating withdrawing treatment as a matter of constitutional right?
4. What are the key differences between the Brother Fox and the John Storar cases?
5. Is the emerging legal consensus described here more restrictive than the ethical position described in chapter 13?

Preview of Chapter 16

- In the battle to resist death, acute care hospitals are sometimes caring for patients who are half-dead.

- Catholic hospitals are committed to "transcendent spiritual beliefs concerning life, suffering, and death."

- Thus, even comatose patients are treated as persons worthy of respect.

- Hospital policies must protect the patient's right to receive ethically ordinary treatment, and preserve the option to forego ethically extraordinary treatment.

- The health care administrator manages the facility through policy and education and relates to various publics.

- Physicians, nurses, and pastoral care persons all have specific roles to play when patient and/or family are considering withdrawing treatment.

CHAPTER 16

Withdrawing Treatment in Catholic Hospitals

In pioneer days it was commonly said of cowboy heroes, "They died with their boots on." Even if their boots were off, it was unlikely that most of the early settlers and pioneers of the United States would die in a hospital.

Times have changed. Approximately 80% of those who die each year in the United States die in an institution. Nursing homes provide an institutional setting for many who die in advanced years. *But over 50% of those who die do so in hospitals today.*[1]

The Battle with Death

Acute care hospitals have become the battleground in the intensive struggle with death. Like modern military battlegrounds, the hospitals

---

[1]Lother, Herman, *Problems of Aging* (Belmont, CA: Dickenson Publ., 1975) p. 138.

overflow with sophisticated electronic and computerized equipment. Like platoon leaders in a military charge, physicians rally their forces for the mortal combat.

In this comparison with warfare, the decision to forego a medical treatment or procedure in a hospital represents a truce with the enemy. For the physician/platoon leader it may seem like surrender. No wonder this complex question generates tension among health care professionals and administrators of health care facilities.

The increasing sophistication and technological efficiency of modern hospitals creates an impression of superiority over the enemy, death. In fact, that efficiency often leads only to a delaying action in the face of the inevitable death. Some writers speak of prolonging biological life but not personal life. Thus, the Anglican Church of Canada Task Force on Human Life makes the statement, "Human life, but not personhood, lingers on until the functions of other body organs fail, often as a result of infection."[2] A case study in a recent book on *Ethical Options in Medicine* by Gregory E. Pence speaks of a comatose grandmother who, "for practical purposes isn't a person, but merely a human body."[3]

Hospitals are caring for human individuals like these who have suffered partial brain death and are irreversibly comatose. In the two quotations just given such individuals are denied the dignity and, presumably, the rights of human persons. What effect will this have on hospital policies and procedures?

As a matter of fact, the very possibility that human individuals might be biologically alive through partial brain function and yet no longer actually be human persons is highly dubious. The whole thrust of the Catholic theology of the person centers on the unity and individuality of each person. Life signs, like heart circulation and respiration (unless artificially simulated), indicate the continued unity of a living human person, even though some brain functions have ceased.

Thus, the comatose grandmother should be considered still a living human person, the same person she was before the coma. To say that human life lingers on, but personhood does not, would mean, in Catholic language, that the soul of the comatose person has left behind a living body in the hospital. Such a novel hypothesis has not been established in science and philosophy and must not be followed in practice.[4]

---

[2]*Dying,* Consideration Concerning the Passage from Life to Death, edited by Lawrence Whytehead and Paul Chidwick (Toronto: The Anglican Book Centre, 1980, p. 45.)

[3]Publ. by Medical Economics Co., Book Division, Oradell, N.J., 1980, p. 66.

[4]See discussion of partial brain death in *Health Care Ethics,* A Theological Analysis, by Benedict M. Ashley O.P. and Kevin D. O'Rourke O.P. (St. Louis, MO: The Catholic Health Association, 1982, Second Edition) pp. 368–369.

Returning to the battlefield comparison described above, the medical war with death today sometimes leaves lying on the battlefield patients like these who seem to be half-dead. To call them merely living bodies and non-persons attacks their inherent dignity and their very identity. The Catholic tradition would reject such language as well as the popular term of "human vegetables," in favor of a more correct and value-rich term, "severely handicapped persons."

Catholic Hospitals

This description of the situation of hospital patients lingering between life and death presents one example of the many challenges facing Catholic hospitals in the United States today. *These hospitals represent by far the largest group of religiously-sponsored hospitals in the nation.* The Catholic Health Association, based in St. Louis, Missouri, represents 633 hospitals, offering nearly 170,000 beds with 6 million admissions per year and nearly 48 million patient days in the last fiscal year.

Catholic hospitals were founded and still exist to provide health care according to Christian ideals and as a reflection of the Catholic Church's concern for suffering and dying persons. Despite tremendous economic challenges, complicated and often burdensome government regulations, and the increasing sophistication and specialization of modern medicine, these hospitals continue to fulfill their mission.

The Preamble to *The Ethical and Religious Directives for Catholic Health Facilities* cites several ideals of Catholic health care facilities: Humble service to humanity and especially to the poor; medical competence and leadership; and fidelity to the Church's teachings while ministering to the good of the whole person.[5] One other ideal applies particularly to the subject of irreversibly comatose persons: "testifying to transcendent spiritual beliefs concerning life, suffering, and death."

The previous three chapters of this volume have discussed the ethical and legal aspects of prolonging life decisions and withdrawing treatment. This chapter will discuss the making of such decisions in Catholic hospitals and, comparably, in Catholic nursing homes. Obviously, *these institutions wish to approach such decisions within the context of the "transcen-*

---

[5]The *Directives* were approved in November, 1971, as the national code, subject to the approval of each bishop for use in his diocese. Copies available from Publications Dept., Catholic Health Association of the United States, 4455 Woodson Road, St. Louis, MO 63134.

dent spiritual beliefs concerning life, suffering, and death" of the Catholic Church.

For example, Catholic health care facilities will manifest their own value-system by careful efforts to avoid terms like "human vegetables" for comatose patients. Furthermore, since they are committed to the stewardship of life tradition and the pro-life ideology mentioned in this volume, they have a definite and clear philosophy about prolonging life decisions.

That philosophy stresses two key concerns: 1) consent of patients or their representatives for giving and withdrawing all treatment, and, 2) responsible determination of when medical procedures may be considered ethically extraordinary and neither ethically nor legally obligatory.[6]

Both of these concerns flow from Christian personalism as understood in the Judeo-Christian tradition and Catholic teaching. In a Catholic health care facility, then, the emphasis will fall on a patient's right to forego certain forms of treatment, not on the ambiguous "right to die." Concerns for genuine patient consent will include equal concerns to make sure that ethically ordinary treatment is not abandoned.

In fact, not only will Catholic health care facilities continue to refuse to permit abortion or euthanasia as part of their medical services, they will also refuse to tolerate prolonging life decisions which involve moral negligence and hence approximate the moral evil of euthanasia.

For example, the Infant Doe case presented in the previous chapter seems to manifest moral negligence in the care of that infant. *A Catholic health care facility which testifies to "transcendent beliefs" about life, suffering, and death is obligated not to tolerate such decisions.* On the other hand, Catholic facilities will be prepared for instances in which it is ethically and legally acceptable for treatment to be withdrawn. The Catholic hospital which originally accepted Karen Quinlan for care seems to have been overly cautious in its administrative stand, as were some of the physicians.[7]

Hence the decade of the 1980s will see Catholic health care facilities striving to reflect the ethical values of the Catholic Christian tradition in their policies on prolonging life decisions. The decisions themselves will undoubtedly become more complex and controversial, and the task of the policy-makers and staffs will become correspondingly more difficult

---

[6]See, *Moral Responsibility in Prolonging Life Decisions*, edited by Donald G. McCarthy and Albert S. Moraczewski O.P., (St. Louis, MO, The Pope John Center, 1981, distributed by Franciscan Herald Press, Chicago), especially p. 246.

[7]*Ibid.*, pp. 153–156.

and challenging. The remainder of this chapter will review the challenges faced by the: administrator, physician, nurse, and pastoral care person.

The Administrator

The board members of each Catholic health facility might be described as the stewards of the facility who delegate to the administrator the power to execute policies which they develop and adopt. The three basic board responsibilities are to maintain the mission of the facility; to conserve the human and financial assets of the facility; and to maintain quality service.

The mission of Catholic health care facilities encompasses the total good of the patient, including his or her spiritual and bodily welfare. Furthermore, since "no patient is an island," to paraphrase a well-known slogan, the patient's family becomes the real "unit of care." It is often suggested that British and European hospitals manifest a fuller appreciation of this family dimension than do United States hospitals.

In decisions about withdrawing treatment, patients who are competent need the advice and support of their families. When the patient is not competent, a family representative normally gives consent in behalf of the patient. Hence the ideal of caring for *the patient and family* becomes particularly important in all these decisions.

The administrator, of course, must try to implement the mission of the facility on behalf of the board. Finding ways of welcoming family involvement in patient care without undermining the good order and efficiency of a facility may require wisdom like Solomon's, but it is worth the effort.

The administrator must also implement the board's policy of conserving assets and maintaining quality care. Ethical questions arise in using prolonging life treatments of dubious benefit to a patient, when full reimbursement is unavailable or when other patients have greater hope of benefit from the same limited resources. If a financial policy of prospective reimbursement in anticipation of treatment replaces the traditional retrospective reimbursement afterwards, greater pressure will be created to limit treatment and hasten discharge.

The care of persons making difficult decisions about withdrawing treatment needs special attention in an acute care hospital. In contrast with the usually routine cooperation of health care persons in routine therapeutic treatment, misunderstandings between staff members and between staff and patient or family and heightened emotional stress weaken the spirit of cooperation and communication.

188

How can an administrator realize the mission ideals of a Catholic facility in the face of these difficulties? *Sister Margaret John Kelly D.C.*, former Vice-President for Mission Services of the Catholic Health Association of the United States, *recommends a double role for the administrator: manager and relator.*

In his/her role as manager, the administrator gives leadership through *education* and *policy*. Obviously, the administrator has little time to act as a teacher or lecturer, but he or she can make sure the right kind of education of staff takes place. In the area of prolonging life decisions this clearly includes ethical and legal aspects of these cases as well as the medical implications. Administrators of Catholic facilities are expected to draw upon the rich Catholic tradition in medical ethics and in the moral aspects of prolonging life traditions. Unfortunately, many versions of secular ethics tend to assume that whatever is legally permissible is ethically acceptable. In the case of Infant Doe, mentioned above, that seems not to have been accurate.

Education, in turn, leads to stated policies within a facility, and the policies then demand continuing education. Policies cannot dictate all aspects of staff behavior but they can set up clear objectives for all to follow. For example, family involvement in prolonging life decisions and staff discussions of difficult situations *with the attending physician* are clear objectives.

The second role of an administrator, that of *relator*, refers to the task of translating and explaining the ministry, not the industry, of Catholic health care to various publics. These include the community of persons directly involved in the health care facility itself as well as the larger civic and church communities in which it operates. In a sense, the administrator becomes a witness person to these publics, testifying to the values which give Catholic health care facilities their unique identity.

The administrator will recognize that prolonging life decisions require prayerful and humble reflection by all who would approach them in a context of faith. Presuming that all cases are clearly covered by legal statutes or precedents can only create a false sense of security and an excuse to overlook relevant ethical principles. Every good administrator watches out for malpractice liability but, *without equal religious and ethical concern, this precautionary outlook becomes a kind of institutional legalism.*

Catholic health care facilities have a proud heritage of quality care and medical excellence, warmly encouraged by the sponsoring religious communities. Administrators are seeking to emphasize the religious origins and character of their facilities. The creative way in which they manage the prolonging life policies and decisions of their facilities and relate to their several publics will enhance that emphasis.

The Physician

The image of a physician/platoon leader directing the battle against death may suggest that physicians generally insist on using every possible medical treatment for their patients. This is surely an exaggeration. Yet some physicians are noted for "never giving up."

In the case of competent patients, physicians must obtain informed consent from them for the treatments they will use. In the case of noncompetent patients, that consent must be given by patient representatives. The ethical principles about giving consent presume that the physician will not bias the discussion either in favor of, or against, further treatment according to the physician's own outlook.

Since Catholic hospitals profess "transcendent spiritual beliefs concerning life, suffering, and death," physicians should find a favorable climate for frank and open discussions of prolonging life decisions. As a matter of policy, Catholic hospitals promote truth-telling to patients. For instance, Directive #8 of the *Ethical and Religious Directives for Catholic Health Facilities* says that:

> Everyone has the right and the duty to prepare for the solemn moment of death. Unless it is clear, therefore, that a dying patient is already well-prepared for death as regards both spiritual and temporal affairs, it is the physician's duty to inform him of his critical condition or to have some other responsible person impart this information.[8]

Physicians become experienced at communicating with patients about terminal illness. Sometimes patients simply refuse to acknowledge what they are told. At other times patients already sense that they are dying, without being told. Even though nurses and pastoral care persons assist greatly in communicating with patients who are terminally ill, the attending physician still holds the primary responsibility.

Two separate steps are always involved in decisions about withdrawing or withholding treatment: a judgment and a decision. First, a *judgment* must be made: Can this treatment be considered ethically optional, does it go beyond a standard of reasonable care? Then, if the judgment is affirmative about the ethical option in this case, a *decision* must be made. The decision may still call for the treatment, even though it is not ethically obligatory. The decision belongs, first of all, to the patient. The judgment does, too, but the physician and health care team must participate in it because of their professional knowledge of the situation.

---

[8]See note 5 above.

The physicians especially need the nurses' knowledge because of their continuing care of the patient during the physicians' absence.

The Nurse

The increasing sophistication of health care treatments and the use of more complex medications and medical equipment have increased the responsibilities of nurses. While the attending physician directs the various therapeutic efforts in the hospital from a distance, the nurse remains on duty for an eight hour shift. The nurse has first-hand knowledge which cannot all be written down on the patient's chart.

This puts the nurse in a mediating position for interaction with both the attending physician and the patient's family. Wise physicians take time to discuss their patients' progress with the nurses on duty. When they do not, both physicians and nurses are handicapped in their work. If the attending physicians neglect to communicate adequately with the nurses, they readily experience frustration.

In these cases, the nurses cannot properly explain to the patient the reasons why the physicians are giving various orders for treatment. The nurses' frustration becomes intense when a decision about withholding or initiating treatment seems dubious and no explanation is offered by the physician. Nurses sometimes feel that their patients' legitimate desire to forego an ethically optional treatment have been ignored. *Because of the Christian commitment to patients' rights and informed consent, Catholic hospitals have a special duty to provide ways of solving such tense situations.*

In chapter 14 of this volume some case studies of prolonging life decisions were presented. For example, Mrs. B. decided to forego further hemodialysis. Undoubtedly, she discussed that decision with the nurses who cared for her long before the physicians set up their formal interview with her. The nurses' knowledge of Mrs. B's judgment about the excess burden of her treatment would be most useful to the physicians in such an interview.

Sometimes, as in the case of Wilhelm K., the nurses seem to know the wishes of the patient more accurately than the family does. Wilhelm apparently wished heroic measures, but his family did not. One kind of heroic measure would be resuscitation after a cardiac arrest. If the attending physician had written an order for no resuscitation, sometimes called a "no-code" order, the nurses would have been obliged *not to call* for the emergency resuscitation team in case Wilhelm had a cardiac arrest.

Nurses more often experience the opposite situation. In such a case, they are caring for a dying patient, but no order has been written to exclude the resuscitation effort. The nurse may be convinced that such a procedure is ethically optional and contrary to the wishes of the dying person. Hospital policies and legal standards demand that a code should be called if a written order does not exclude it. Nurses in these cases are tempted to walk slowly to the phone. Someone called this the "shuffling of the feet" syndrome. Good hospital policy would insist that physicians consider writing the "no-code" order in appropriate cases and after consultation with the patient and family.

Nurses, therapists, and even hospital housekeepers get to know the patients in a more personal way than many physicians do. That is why they have a necessary role in decisions to withdraw treatment. Another member of the health care team, the pastoral care person, comes to know the patient from a new and important perspective.

The Pastoral Care Person

During the years of renewal in the Catholic Church since the Second Vatican Council ended in 1965, a parallel renewal has occurred in the pastoral care ministry of Catholic hospitals. The Sacraments of Anointing, Holy Eucharist, and Reconciliation are administered in English, instead of Latin, with increased understanding and participation by those receiving them. Pastoral care staffs have expanded to include, besides Catholic priests, women and men of religious communities, ministers of other religious traditions, and trained lay persons.

These pastoral care persons have learned to listen to the verbal and non-verbal communication of patients and their families. Their assistance and active involvement with health care professionals in the difficult cases of withdrawing or withholding treatment can bring great comfort to patients and their families.

Also, pastoral care persons often become the "resident experts" in hospitals on the ethical principles about prolonging life. Chapter 20 of the Pope John Center resource book, *Moral Responsibility in Prolonging Life Decisions,* discusses their role more fully.[9] Pastoral care persons bring a faith perspective to these situations. At times when a truce should be concluded in the medical battle with death, the pastoral care persons must carry the responsibility of peace-maker and reconciler. Catholic hospitals are expected to have equal competence in resisting suffering and death and in assisting patients when the time has come to accept death.

---

[9]*Op. cit.* in #6 above, pp. 279–289.

Discussion Questions

1. Why is health care like a military battle?
2. In the light of the personalism presented in this volume, why should irreversibly comatose persons still be considered living persons?
3. How could a hospital avoid permitting a case like that of Infant Doe to occur in its facility?
4. How should a health care facility go about formulating its policies about withdrawing treatment?
5. What is the difference between the judgment and the decision in cases of withdrawing treatment?
6. Discuss the mediating roles of nurses and pastoral care persons.

Preview of Chapter 17

- Up until recent times death was recognized by the cessation of spontaneous breathing and pulse.

- Now artificial procedures can maintain breathing and pulse although the patient may actually have died.

- Brain-related criteria have been developed by the medical profession to indicate the total and irreversible cessation of all brain functions, including the brain stem.

- Brain activity is essential to the unifying of activity in the human organism and to human life itself.

- Hence, although some disagreement exists about the reliability of various sets of brain-related criteria for death, when a person has undergone true and total brain death, the person is dead.

- The need for state statutes permitting determination of death by brain-related criteria is disputed.

CHAPTER 17

Determining Death by Brain Criteria

Introduction

Not least among the life and death issues is the question, "Just when is a person dead?" A few years ago, a young man fell into the icy waters of Lake Michigan near Chicago. It was estimated that he had been under the water for approximately 22 minutes. When he was finally pulled out by a rescue team, there were no signs of life: no detectable respiration, no noticeable heartbeat, his skin color was gray and, apparently, there was no response to any kind of vocal or other stimuli.

The rescue team decided that the individual was dead and was carrying him back to the ambulance when suddenly he coughed, or gasped, which caught the attention of the stretcher bearers. They uncovered him and began cardiopulmonary resuscitation. After two hours he began to breath on his own and the pulse was firm. He was then taken to a hospital where he received further treatment. After a few weeks he was released from the hospital with no apparent damage—

physical or psychological—resulting from his experience. He went back to college and earned straight A's.

Many people fear that they may be treated as dead—even buried—while they are alive. With the modern practice of embalming, however, this is not very likely to occur.

People also fear being kept "alive" by extreme measures after they are medically dead. The concern here is primarily for the impact such treatment would have on their friends and relatives since the individuals would actually be dead.

Death in Former Years

Until very recent times, that is, until the last 25 years or so, death was recognized simply by the cessation of spontaneous breathing and pulse over a certain amount of time, perhaps 30 minutes. The doctor checked the individual's respiration and heartbeat and looked at the pupils to see whether they were fixed and dilated. If the individual was not responsive to stimuli, and respiration and pulse was absent, the doctor would then simply inform the family and/or bystanders that the individual was dead.

The process of determining death seemed rather uncomplicated and quite certain. While in some cultures it was necessary to bury the individual before sundown, in our culture the body was ordinarily transferred to the morgue and embalmed. Certainly, if the individual had not died before, he would have died there and then as a result of the embalming. After the body underwent rigor mortis there was no doubt in anyone's mind that the individual was certainly dead.

Death Today

Because of advances in biomedical technology, the means are available for providing life support for any individual whose vital systems are functioning at a minimal level or not at all. There are artificial respirators that can maintain respiration in an individual. Circulation can be restored by electrical stimulation or by chemical means which are effective in restoring and, in many instances, maintaining an adequate heartbeat and circulation.

As a consequence of these abilities to provide life support, serious problems arise in the legal handling of homicides, negligence claims, insurance questions, the transplantation of anatomical parts, workers'

196

compensation, probate law and taxes. Consider a person who is hit by an automobile, brought to the emergency room, and put on artificial life-support systems. If that patient dies before these systems are turned off, it is difficult to determine the time of death: Was it at the time of the accident or at some later point?

Associated with the ability to restore or maintain respiration and circulation by artificial means are several important ethical and theological questions. Certainly, because of our common reverence for life, *it is morally unacceptable to terminate a person's life by declaring him or her dead before the individual is actually deceased.* There are certain groups and individuals today who are seeking to legalize the possibility of pronouncing persons clinically dead before they are really dead. Consequently, it is important that the determination of death be made by objectively verifiable criteria that are accurate, practical and reliable.

On the other side of the coin, there is a concern that, when appropriate, persons be able to donate their organs for the benefit of others. The problem that arises here is one of pinpointing, as closely as possible, the exact moment when the donor dies. Organs deteriorate rapidly after death; waiting too long will render them useless for transplantation. On the other hand, because pressure to retrieve them in usable condition is often extreme, medical personnel must be careful to assure that the potential donor is truly dead before removing any organs.

When a person is being maintained on a life-support system, it is difficult to determine whether spontaneous respiration is present or absent. Because the customary methods of determining death are difficult to apply when the person is on life-support systems, other criteria have evolved in the last 25 years. These criteria are related to the brain, and variously referred to as brain death criteria, or brain-related criteria. They have been accepted by the majority of the medical profession and have entered the legal field by incorporation into the determination-of-death statutes passed by some states.

Uniform Determination of Death Act

As a consequence of the many discussions among physicians and employers and others, a variety of proposals have been made for criteria to be used for the determination of death. After more than a dozen years of discussion, a model statute has been proposed and has been accepted by the American Bar Association and the American Medical Association. It reads as follows:

An individual who has sustained either 1) the irreversible cessation of circulatory and respiratory functions, or 2) the irreversible cessation of all functions of the entire brain, including the brain stem, is dead. A determination of death must be made in accordance with accepted medical standards.[1]

The burden of this chapter will be to discuss the theological and ethical dimensions of that definition relative to Christian values.

The nature of the human person and the sanctity of human life have been discussed in earlier chapters of this book; they will not be repeated here. For a Catholic, any analysis of death has to keep in mind the teachings of the Church regarding life and death. For a Christian, death is not seen as a total destruction or annihilation of the human person. Rather, it is a transition to eternal life.

One should recall that the human person is a composite of matter and spirit. It is neither the body nor the soul, but the composite which forms a single living, existing thing, the human person. At death, the individual enters into a different mode of existence. But the human person continues to exist as an individual after death.

Death, then, can be viewed from two different perspectives, death as disintegration and death as transformation. *Death as disintegration* is what we witness and experience: Shortly after death the body begins to disintegrate, fall apart. We refer to that event by saying that the soul leaves the body. What "leaving" the body precisely means is not known. However, once the event occurs, the body no longer is a unified being; it begins immediately but gradually to fall apart into its respective components.

On the other hand, *death as transformation* is not in itself a painful process but rather a transition from one mode of existence to another. This means that the human person existing on this earth here and now, in time and space, without losing continuity of existence, enters into another mode of existence which is eternal, and transcends the limitations of time and space as we now experience them. Consequently, when we look at death, we are not witnessing the termination of a person but rather the transformation of a person from one life to another life.

Medical and Scientific Dimensions

By what process is a person declared dead by a physician? The physician determines that death has occurred by certain signs; classically,

---

[1]"Guidelines for the Determination of Death." *Journal of the American Medical Association*, Vol. 246, No. 19, pp. 2184–86.

these have been the end of spontaneous breathing and heartbeat. Physicians know from personal experience as well as experience built up over many years by the medical community that respiration and heartbeat do not ordinarily start again spontaneously after they have ceased for a certain period of time.

Respiration and heartbeat are chosen as indicators of life and death because of their central functions in the maintenance of the body's survival. The function of respiration, breathing, is for the purpose of bringing oxygen from the outside and allowing it to enter into the blood stream. At the same time, the blood stream gives up the carbon dioxide which has accumulated from the metabolic activity of the cells. The function of the heart as a pump is basically to maintain the blood circulation through all the parts of the body, so that with the help of blood vessels—arteries, veins, and capillaries—the blood reaches every part of the body carrying the oxygen which the living cells need so desperately. When a cell, or tissue, or organ does not receive sufficient oxygen, or no oxygen at all for a matter of relatively a few minutes, 15–20 minutes, the cells, tissues, or organs are so damaged that they never recover: that is, they have died. When the entire brain in particular has undergone such a truly irreversible cessation of activity, we can say that the individual is dead.

The death of the individual, it should be carefully noted, is not associated with any particular cells, tissues or organs *as such*. A person can lose a leg, arm or have a kidney removed or become blind and deaf, and so on, without being dead. Death, rather, is the cessation of the individual as a whole, the human organism as a unit is no longer a unit and functioning. This is where the brain has an essential and unique role.

Over the years, medical and biological sciences have discovered that the brain (and the rest of the central nervous system) are essential to the unifying activity of the human organism. It seems that every effort of the body is made to maintain the brain in functioning order. Food is brought to the body through the mouth in order that energy be available for the brain to function. Muscles are used to bring the body to food. The bones are necessary to give the body a certain rigidity and structure in order for it to move, and the skull protects the brain from injury.

The blood is directed towards maintaining circulation, not only to keep the other organs alive, but especially to keep the brain alive. In moments of crisis, for example, a person might faint; the body falls down in order to restore the blood pressure in the brain and thus meet a dangerous situation where the blood pressure has dropped in the brain. When there is a great loss of blood, circulation is shut down to some parts of the body, but maintained to the brain and the heart. In other words, it seems that every effort of the body's tissues and organs is directed ultimately to maintain the brain in functioning order.

If the brain is fully deprived of oxygen for 8 to 10 minutes, it becomes so damaged that it cannot recover. This is true, however, only at or near normal body temperature. If the body temperature drops only 7 to 10 degrees, then the brain's need for oxygen is decreased and it can stand the absence of oxygen for a longer period of time. *This fact is a likely explanation of what happened with the young man who had fallen into the ice cold waters of Lake Michigan and yet survived as was recounted at the beginning of this chapter.*

Does that mean that death of the brain is the same thing as death of the individual? As noted above, care must be taken not to *identify* any one organ or one part of the body with the person. The person is the entire human organism. Any part of the body is part of the human person because it is animated and unified by the one soul. While it is true that the basic source of unity of the living being is the soul, it is also true that the unifying power is exercised primarily by means of the brain or central nervous system, and only secondarily by the hormonal and, to some extent, the circulatory system.

However, cessation of spontaneous respiration and circulation are the traditional methods of determining death because they indicate that the brain has died. While the heart can go on beating without input from the central nervous system, spontaneous respiration depends for its activity on a part of the brain found in the brain stem. Should that part be destroyed, or in other ways impeded from acting, then respiration will not proceed.

Death of the brain can be clinically determined by a number of signs, such as a deep unresponsive coma; fixed and dilated pupils; loss of spontaneous breathing; absence of certain reflexes; and a "flat" EEG and/or cessation of brain-blood flow for at least 20 to 30 minutes. It is very important that the cause of the coma which could account for the observed loss of brain function be determined, because some of these signs can be mimicked by other conditions. Shock, low body temperature, and presence of certain central nervous system depressant drugs in the body are factors that must be taken into account in making the determination of brain death.

A cautionary note needs to be introduced, irreversible *coma* is *not* brain death or death. In such a condition the brain stem, at the very least, is still functioning.

Given our present scientific data and a coherent rational analysis of it, we are at the present time obliged morally at least to *presume* that *an individual in an irreversible coma is still alive until all brain functions, including brain stem function, irreversibly cease.*

200

The ability to maintain respiration with a mechanical ventilator, and circulation with the aid of drugs, creates ethical and psychological problems. It is difficult to believe that a person is dead when the patient appears to be breathing, and has skin which is soft and warm. To all superficial appearances, the person appears to be alive; yet, by brain-related criteria, the physician would say the person is dead. It is known from experience that once the brain has died, then these artificial support systems are only effective for a matter of a few days, or weeks at the most. Eventually the whole system breaks down and no effort made can continue respiration and circulation.

It is the position of the editors of this book that a person who has undergone true brain death as defined above is really dead. Even though respiration, heart action, and circulation could be maintained by certain means for a while in such a brain-dead individual, the person is dead because there is no longer a truly unified being. There are no *human* organs or human *person;* the individual has now entered into another mode of existence. What we observe in this body is merely the *appearance* of life. Remove these life support systems and everything comes to a grinding halt.

Legal Aspects of Determination of Death By Brain Criteria

At the time of this writing some 30 states have laws to permit determination of death by brain related criteria.[2] The actual wording varies from state to state; further, some of the laws are more open than others to misapplication or abuse.

The various state statutes regarding brain related criteria for the determination of death can be grouped for convenience into three types: (1) those which offer alternative definitions; (2) those which are applicable only when the use of artificial life support systems would interfere with the determination of death by the traditional means; and (3) those in which only the brain-related criteria are mentioned.

An example of the first type is the Kansas statute which, in 1970, was the first such legislation to be enacted:

A person will be considered medically and legally dead if, in the opinion of a physician, based on ordinary standards of medical practice, there is the absence of spontaneous respiratory and cardiac func-

---

[2]Most of this subject material can be found in, *Determination of Death,* edited by Albert S. Moraczewski, O.P., and J. Stuart Showalter (St. Louis, MO, The Catholic Health Association of the U.S., 1982), pp. 21–30.

tion and, because of the disease or condition which caused, directly or indirectly, these functions to cease, or because of the passage of time since these functions ceased, attempts at resuscitation are considered hopeless; and, in this event, death will have occurred at the time these functions ceased; or

A person will be considered medically and legally dead if, in the opinion of a physician, based on ordinary standards of medical practice, there is the absence of spontaneous brain function; and if based on ordinary standards of medical practice, during reasonable attempts to either maintain or restore spontaneous circulatory or respiratory function in the absence of aforesaid brain function, it appears that further attempts at resuscitation or supportive maintenance will not succeed, death will have occurred at the time when these conditions first coincide. Death is to be pronounced before any vital organ is removed for purposes of transplantation.

These alternative definitions of death are to be utilized for all purposes in this state, including the trials of civil and criminal cases, any laws to the contrary notwithstanding.

The statute passed by the State of Michigan is an example of the second type:

A person will be considered dead if, in the announced opinion of a physician, based on ordinary standards of medical practice in the community, there is the irreversible cessation of spontaneous respiratory and circulatory function. If artificial means of support preclude a determination that these functions have ceased, a person will be considered dead if in the announced opinion of a physician, based on ordinary standards of medical practice in the community, there is the irreversible cessation of spontaneous brain function. Death will have occurred at the time when the relevant functions ceased. (Emphasis added.)

The third group may be represented by the Georgia statute:

A person may be pronounced dead if it is determined that the person has suffered an irreversible cessation of brain function. There shall be independent confirmation of the death by another physician.

As noted above, about three-fifths of the states have to date adopted some statutory form of determination of death by brain related criteria. Of those who have not, some have adopted such a definition in case law.

The Supreme Court of Arizona, for example, in *State v. Fierro* did just that. In this case, the defendant had argued that there was insufficient basis to convict him of murder by gunshot because his victim died only after being removed from systems. The Supreme Court disagreed:

> *The removal of the life support systems was not the proximate cause of death, the gunshot wounds were, and it was not error to find that the defendant was the cause of the victim's death.*
>
> *We also believe that the defendant was legally dead before the life support systems were withdrawn . . . [O]ur legislature . . . has not adopted a definition of death. A statutory definition is not necessary, however.*
>
> *We believe that while the common law definition of death is still sufficient to establish death, [brain death] is properly supported by expert medical testimony, and is also a valid test for death in Arizona.*

In addition to these various legislative and court actions, the legal "bible," *Black's Law Dictionary* in its new Fifth Edition, includes the concept of brain death:

> **Brain death.** Numerous states have enacted statutory definitions of death which include brain-related criteria. "A person shall be pronounced dead if it is determined by a physician that the person has suffered a total and irreversible cessation of brain function. There shall be independent confirmation of the death by another physician." Calif. Health & Safety Code, Section 7180 (1976).
>
> *Characteristics of brain death consist of: (1) unreceptivity and unresponsiveness to externally applied stimuli and internal needs; (2) no spontaneous movements or breathing; (3) no reflex activity; and (4) a flat electroencephalograph reading after 24 hours period of observation. Com. v. Golston, Mass., 366 N.E. 2d 744. An increasing number of states have adopted this so-called "Harvard" definition of brain death, either by statute or court decision.*
>
> **Death.** The cessation of life; permanent cessations of all vital functions and signs. Numerous states have enacted statutory definitions of death which include brain-related criteria.[3]

---

[3]*Black's Law Dictionary*, 170, 360 (5th Ed. 1979).

A major conference at Vanderbilt University, aided by new diagnostic neurological testing, considered some of the philosophical and legal aspects of whole-brain, neocortical, and higher brain criteria.[4] It is precisely this kind of scientific data that is needed for further precise ethical evaluation.

Concern has been expressed that the existence of brain-death statutes on the books might promote or prepare the way for legally approved euthanasia (mercy killing). Others feel that brain death legislation is necessary in order to prevent the courts from arbitrary actions or from accepting a definition of death which would not be adequate from a Christian perspective. While one cannot foresee all the possible abuses that can arise from a particular piece of legislation, it is important that an informed public be aware of what are the possibilities in order to intervene in an appropriate manner when so indicated.

Discussion Questions

1. Do you think the young man in Lake Michigan was actually dead and came alive again?
2. What are the moral implications of declaring someone dead when they are not actually deceased?
3. What is the significance of the model statute on determination of death accepted by the American Bar Association and the American Medical Association?
4. What do you mean by death as *disintegration* and death as *transformation*?
5. What causes brain cells to die?
6. What is the difference between death and irreversible coma? What are some signs of death of the brain?

---

[4]*Death: Beyond Whole-Brain Criteria*, edited by Richard M. Zaner (Boston: Kluwer Academic Publishers, 1988).

Bibliography

The following books offer further resource material on the themes of this
Handbook. *They are selected as representative of the Judeo-Christian tradition
and Catholic teaching.*

Ashley, O.P., Benedict M. and O'Rourke O.P., Kevin D. **Health Care Ethics, A Theologi-
cal Analysis.** St. Louis, MO: Catholic Health Assoc. of the U.S., 2nd Edit., 1982.
Connery, S.J., John R. **Abortion: The Development of the Roman Catholic Perspective.**
Chicago, IL: Loyola University Press, 1977.
Death, Dying and Euthanasia, edited by Dennis J. Horan and David Mall. Washington,
D. C.: University Publications of America, 1977.
An Ethical Evaluation of Fetal Experimentation: An Interdisciplinary Study, edited by
Donald G. McCarthy and Albert S. Moraczewski O.P. St. Louis, MO: The Pope John
Center, 1976.
Grisez, Germain, **Abortion: the Myths, the Realities, and the Arguments.** New York: Cor-
pus Books, 1970.
Grisez, Germain, and Boyle, Joseph M. **Life and Death with Liberty and Justice: A Con-
tribution to the Euthanasia Debate.** Notre Dame, IN: University of Notre Dame
Press, 1979.
Lamerton, Richard. **Care for the Dying.** Gretna, LA: Pelican Press, 1981.
Mall, David and Watts, Walter F., M.D., **The Psychological Effects of Abortion.** Washing-
ton, D.C.: University Publications of America, 1979.
May, William E. **Human Existence, Medicine, and Ethics.** Chicago, IL: Franciscan Herald
Press, 1977.
May, William E. and Westley, Richard. **The Right to Die.** Chicago, IL, Thomas More
Press, 1980.
McFadden, O.S.A., Charles J. **The Dignity of Life.** Huntington, IN: Our Sunday Visitor
Press, 1976.
Moraczewski O.P., Albert S. and Showalter, J. Stuart. **Determination of Death,** Theologi-
cal, Medical, Ethical and Legal Issues. St. Louis, MO: The Catholic Hospital Assoc. of
U.S., 1982.
Moral Responsibility in Prolonging Life Decisions, edited by Donald G. McCarthy and
Albert S. Moraczewski O.P. St. Louis, MO: The Pope John Center; distributed by
Franciscan Herald Press, Chicago, 1981.
Nathanson, Bernard N. and Ostling, Richard N. **Aborting America.** Garden City, N.Y.:
Doubleday & Co., 1979.

Nelson, J. Robert, **Science and Our Troubled Conscience.** Philadelphia: Fortress Press, 1980.

New Perspectives on Human Abortion, edited by Thomas W. Hilgers, Dennis J. Horan, and David Mall. Frederick, MD.: University Publications of America, 1981.

New Technologies of Birth and Death. St. Louis, MO: The Pope John Center, distributed by Franciscan Herald Press, Chicago, IL, 1980.

Noonan, John T. **A Private Choice, Abortion in America in the Seventies.** New York: The Free Press, 1979.

Powell, S.J., John. **Abortion: The Silent Holocaust.** Niles, IL: Argus Communications, 1981.

Principles of Catholic Theology, A Synthesis of Dogma and Morals, edited by Edward Gratsch. Staten Island, N.Y.: Alba House, 1981.

Ramsey, Paul. **Ethics at the Edges of Life.** New Haven, CT: Yale University Press, 1978.

Schaeffer, Francis A., and Koop, C. Everett, M.D. **Whatever Happened to the Human Race?** Old Tappan, N.J.: Fleming H. Revell Co., 1979.

Weber, Leonard J. **Who Shall Live?** The Dilemma of Severely Handicapped Children and Its Meaning for Other Moral Questions. New York: Paulist Press, 1976.

Pope John Center Publications

The Pope John XXIII Medical-Moral Research and Education Center has dedicated itself to approaching current and emerging medical-moral issues from the perspective of Catholic teaching and the Judeo-Christian heritage. Publications of the Pope John Center include:

REPRODUCTIVE TECHNOLOGIES, MARRIAGE AND THE CHURCH (Proceedings of the 1988 Bishops' Workshop), 318 pp., $17.95.
This book provides a commentary on and a discussion of the Vatican's *Instruction on Respect for Human Life in its Origin and on the Dignity of Procreation* (1987). Topics covered range from an overview of current magisterial teaching regarding procreation to a consideration of the values presupposed by reproductive technologies, an update on AIDS, and suggestions for pastoral applications of the Church's teaching on human procreation and sexual diseases.

CRITICAL ISSUES IN CONTEMPORARY HEALTH CARE (Proceedings of the 1989 Bishops' Workshop). Edited by Russell E. Smith. $17.95.
This book centers around the general theme of health care and its technologies. Among the specific topics treated are: euthanasia, the right to die movements, pastoral considerations of life and death issues, ethics committees in health care facilities, fetal and newborn tissue transplants, psychosexual maturity, Catholic identity and hospital mergers, moral issues in the artificial provision of nutrition and hydration, and teaching moral theology in the comtemporary world.

THE AIDS CRISIS AND THE CONTRACEPTIVE MENTALITY by Msgr. Orville N. Griese, S.T.D., J.C.D., and Dr. Eugene F. Diamond with a Pastoral Commentary by The Most Reverend Donald W. Montrose, 1988, 69 pp., $3.95.
A moral evaluation of potential means of protecting the general population from the scourge of AIDS . . . Using the AIDS crisis to renew dedication to Christian standards of morality.

SEXUALITY: THEOLOGICAL VOICES—Kevin T. McMahon $14.95.
A Critical Analysis of American Catholic Theological Thought from 1965 through 1980.

THEOLOGIANS AND AUTHORITY WITHIN THE LIVING CHURCH by Msgr. James J. Mulligan, 1986, 139 pp., $13.95.
The author's intention is to answer some questions that have been raised about the proper place of authority and theology in the Catholic Thurch. Using clear and readable language, the author seeks to explain, to clarify and to share with the reader a context within which he thinks there can be peace.

CATHOLIC IDENTITY IN HEALTH CARE By Msgr. Orville N. Griese, S.T.D., J.C.D., 1987, 537 pp., $17.95.
This book is a detailed commentary on the *Ethical and Religious Di-*

rectives for Catholic Health Facilities approved by the National Conference of Catholic Bishops. The author organized his material around nine core principles upon which the *Directives* **rest.**

SCARCE MEDICAL RESOURCES AND JUSTICE (Proceedings of the 1987 Bishops' Workshop). $17.95.
These are the Proceedings of the 1987 Bishops' Workshop in which, with the help of appropriate experts, the bishops pondered the respective responsibilities of individuals and various institutions with regards to the equitable distribution of burdens and benefits in the provision of health care.

CONSERVING HUMAN LIFE (The Pope John Center Edition) by The Most Reverend Daniel A. Cronin, $13.95.
Originally written in 1958 before the issue had become emotionally charged, this updated and edited version of a doctoral dissertation traces the development of the Church's understanding of the moral law in regard to the ordinary and extraordinary means of conserving life. With Commentaries. 1989

THE FAMILY TODAY AND TOMORROW: The Church Addresses Her Future (proceedings of the 1985 Bishops' Workshop) Edited by Donald G. McCarthy, Ph.D., 1985, 291 pp., $17.95.
One of the family's fundamental tasks is: "to build up the kingdom of God in history by participating in the life and mission of the Church" (Familiaris Consortio, 49). The challenges and obstacles that inhibit the family in this role today are examined, with reflections from the Church's teachings and possible future directions. Fifteen experts in sociology, psychology, medicine and theology have contributed to this volume.

THEOLOGIES OF THE BODY: Humanist and Christian By Benedict M. Ashley, O.P., 1985, 770 pp., $20.95.
With a rare breadth of vision and insightful erudition, this wide ranging theological study of human materiality compares and contrasts two world viewpoints—the humanist and the Christian. It is an historical, philosophical and theological approach to a non-dualistic anthropology as a foundation for Christian ethics.

MORAL THEOLOGY TODAY: Certitudes and Doubts (Proceedings of the 1984 Bishops' Workshop) 1984, 355 pp., $17.95.
This book presents a concise survey of morals and ethics in their biblical and systematic theology roots, their historical development, and the relationships of theologians to bishops, the tradition and the magisterium. Contemporary challenges in moral methodologies are examined and compared with traditional principles of exceptionless moral norms, totality, double-effect and the moral inseparability of the unitive and procreative meanings of the conjugal act.

SEX AND GENDER: A Theological and Scientific Inquiry Edited by Mark Schwartz, Sc.D., Albert S. Moraczewski, OP, Ph.D. and James A. Monteleone, MD, 1983, 385 pp., $19.95.
This is an attempt to provide in the area of human sexuality the most current scientific data and additional psychological, philosoph-

ical and theological reflections upon that data from the viewpoint of the meanings of sexuality as expressed in Catholic teaching.

TECHNOLOGICAL POWERS AND THE PERSON: Nuclear Energy and Reproductive Technologies (Proceedings of the 1983 Bishops' Workshop) 1983, 500 pp., $15.95.
In the 1983 Dallas workshop, the assembled bishops listened, pondered and reacted to scientific and theological experts speaking on the awesome powers of nuclear energy (for peaceful purposes) and reproductive technologies. This book is a collection of the lectures and edited discussions.

HANDBOOK ON CRITICAL SEXUAL ISSUES Edited by Donald G. McCarthy, Ph.D. and Edward J. Bayer, S. T. D. Revised edition, 1989. 230 pp., $9.95.
Taking an historical approach beginning with biblical roots of Catholic teaching developing through early and medieval periods and bringing it up to post Vatican II, the book attempts to present the roots of sexual norms in Catholic sexual teaching. After discussing the Christian vocation of marriage and natural family planning, the book enters into the second part in which specific sexual issues are considered.

HANDBOOK ON CRITICAL LIFE ISSUES Edited by Donald G. McCarthy, Ph.D. and Edward J. Bayer, S.T.D. Revised edition, 1989. 220 pp., $9.95.
This is a carefully edited version of the presentation made by thirty-one experts in medicine, theology, psychology, law and sociology who for twelve days addressed such issues as abortion, defective fetal development, organ transplants, technology for prolongation of life, and brain-related criterion for the determination of a person's death.

MORAL RESPONSIBILITY IN PROLONGING LIFE DECISIONS Edited by Donald G. McCarthy, Ph.D. and Albert S. Moraczewski, OP, Ph.D., 1982, 316 pp., $9.95.
This book contains twenty chapters plus two appendices and discusses the medical, moral and legal aspects of prolonging life decisions. It also examines the specific responsibilities of administrators of health care facilities, physicians, nurses and pastoral care persons.

HUMAN SEXUALITY AND PERSONHOOD (Proceedings of the 1981 Bishops' Workshop) 1981, 254 pp., $9.95.
With input from several relevant scientific disciplines, this Bishops' Workshop sought to present a contemporary and balanced theology of human sexuality and marriage in the light of magisterial teaching and a Christian theology of the human person.

GENETIC COUNSELING: The Church and the Law Edited by Gary Atkinson, Ph.D. and Albert S. Moraczewski, OP, Ph.D., 1980, 259 pp., $9.95.
An appreciative review in the December 1980 issue of *Theological Studies* (Page 805) describes succinctly: "Highly recommended for genetic counselors, pastors, and students. Its clear common succinct

style makes the book a good introduction to biogenetic morality and a valuable survey of the present debate."

NEW TECHNOLOGIES OF BIRTH AND DEATH: Medical, Legal, and Moral Dimensions (Proceedings of the 1980 Bishop's Workshop) 1980, 196 pp., $8.95.

Five theologians, two physicians and two lawyers discuss subjects as old as abortion and contraception and as new as in vitro fertilization and the ovulation method of family planning. The book also reviews efforts to determine if human death has occurred even though vital signs are artificially maintained.

A MORAL EVALUATION OF CONTRACEPTION AND STERILIZATION: A Dialogical Study by Gary Atkinson, Ph.D. and Albert S. Moraczewski, OP, Ph.D., 1980, 115 pp., $4.95.

The authors of this paper hope it will be a contribution to a more clear understanding of the multifaceted issues of contraception by presenting accurately, clearly, and fairly the principal arguments of this controversy.

ARTFUL CHILDMAKING: Artificial Insemination in Catholic Teaching by John C. Wakefield, Ph.D., 1978, 205 pp., $8.95.

By providing an historical and theological review of the Church's teaching with regard to artificial insemination, the present publication does some of the ground work for an understanding of the Catholic Church's position with regards to technological reproduction.

AN ETHICAL EVALUATION OF FETAL EXPERIMENTATION Edited by Donald G. McCarthy, Ph.D. and Albert S. Moraczewski, OP, Ph.D., 1976, 137 pp., $8.95.

The present study seeks to analyze the ethical issues involved in fetal experimentation and to discover the valid foundations for a broadly based consensus concerning our need as a human, civilized community to protect the fetus. The book also includes a detailed discussion of the issue of delayed hominization and its refutation.

The following books have been published collaboratively with the Catholic Health Association of the United States:

GENETIC MEDICINE AND ENGINEERING: Ethical and Social Dimensions Edited by Albert S. Moraczewski, OP, Ph.D., 1983, 198 pp., $17.50.

This book intends to assist the decision-makers in Catholic Health Ministries, especially in forming appropriate and practical policies in matters concerning these developing technologies in the area of genetic medicine and engineering. It is a collection of articles by experts in the field of genetics and ethics.

ETHICS COMMITTEES: A Challenge for Catholic Health Care Edited by Sister Margaret John Kelly, D.C., Ph.D. and Donald G. McCarthy, Ph.D., 1984, 151 pp., $15.50.

This work treats the various needs which have contributed to the development of the Ethics Committees; reflect on ethical methodologies and legal aspects of such committees and offers models for various types of ethics committees to meet the needs at the institutional, diocesan and multi-institutional system levels.

DETERMINATION OF DEATH: Theological, Medical, Ethical and Legal Issues by Albert S. Moraczewski, OP, Ph.D. and J. Stuart Showalter, JD, MFS, St. Louis, The Catholic Health Association of the U.S. 1982, 39 pp., $2.50.

In a concise manner, this work focuses on the question, "Is the Patient Dead?" In the first section, the biblical and theological roots of the concept of person and the philosophical aspects of life and death are briefly reviewed. In the final section, the statutory and case law aspects are discussed.

As a service to those interested in the meaning of "moral" laws and norms, The Pope John Center is making available a published doctoral dissertation:

THE MEANING OF THE TERM "MORAL" IN ST. THOMAS AQUINAS By Brian Thomas Mullady, OP, S. T. D, Pontifical Academy of St. Thomas, 1986, 142 pp., $12.00.

This work, while probing the meaning of the term moral as used by St. Thomas, looks squarely at some of the contemporary issues especially with regards to the denial of exceptionless moral norms.

These books may be ordered from: The Pope John Center, 186 Forbes Road, Braintree, MA 02184, Telephone (617) 848–6965. Prepayment is encouraged. Please add $1.00 for shipping and handling for the first book ordered and 25 cents for each additional book.

Subscriptions to the Pope John Center monthly newsletter, *ETHICS AND MEDICS,* may be sent to the same address.

Index

War, 37
Ward, Russel, 56
Washington (state), 105
Watergate scandal, 30
Wellness programs, 31–34
Wertham, Fredric, 142
Westberg, Granger, 32–34
Westberg, Jill, 33
White, Justine, 106
Wholeness (person), 15, 62, 67
Wholistic Health Centers, 32

Wholistic medicine, 162–163
Will (human), 15, 19, 40, 113
Wisdom literature, 65
Withdrawal (treatment), 171–182
World Health Organization, 30
Worth, 40

Zalba, Marcello, 92, 129, 130
Zimbardo, Philip, 6
Zygote, 85